**Critical Issues in
Health Policy**

Critical Issues in Health Policy

Edited by

Ralph A. Straetz
New York University

Marvin Lieberman
New York Academy of Medicine

Alice Sardell
Queens College

LexingtonBooks
D.C. Heath and Company
Lexington, Massachusetts
Toronto

Library of Congress Cataloging in Publication Data

Main entry under title:

Critical issues in health policy.

Includes index.
1. Medical policy—United States. 2. Medical policy. I. Straetz, Ralph
Arthur. II. Lieberman, Marvin. III. Sardell, Alice. [DNLM: 1. Health
policy—United States. WA 540 AA1 C9]
RA395.A3C84   362.1'0973   80-9015
ISBN 0-669-04504-7   AACR2

Published simultaneously in Canada

Printed in the United States of America

International Standard Book Number: 0-669-04504-7

Library of Congress Catalog Card Number: 80-9015

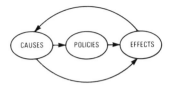

Policy Studies Organization Series

General Approaches to Policy Studies

v

Specific Policy Problems

Analyzing Poverty Policy
  edited by Dorothy Buckton James
Crime and Criminal Justice
  edited by John A. Gardiner and Michael Mulkey
Civil Liberties
  edited by Stephen L. Wasby
Foreign Policy Analysis
  edited by Richard L. Merritt
Economic Regulatory Policies
  edited by James E. Anderson
Political Science and School Politics
  edited by Samuel K. Gove and Frederick M. Wirt
Science and Technology Policy
  edited by Joseph Haberer
Population Policy Analysis
  edited by Michael E. Kraft and Mark Schneider
The New Politics of Food
  edited by Don F. Hadwiger and William P. Browne
New Dimensions to Energy Policy
  edited by Robert Lawrence
Race, Sex, and Policy Problems
  edited by Marian Lief Palley and Michael Preston
American Security Policy and Policy-Making
  edited by Robert Harkavy and Edward Kolodziej
Current Issues in Transportation Policy
  edited by Alan Altshuler
Security Policies of Developing Countries
  edited by Edward Kolodziej and Robert Harkavy
Determinants of Law-Enforcement Policies
  edited by Fred A. Meyer, Jr., and Ralph Baker
Evaluating Alternative Law-Enforcement Policies
  edited by Ralph Baker and Fred A. Meyer, Jr.
International Energy Policy
  edited by Robert M. Lawrence and Martin O. Heisler
Employment and Labor-Relations Policy
  edited by Charles Bulmer and John L. Carmichael, Jr.
Housing Policy for the 1980s
  edited by Roger Montgomery and Dale Rogers Marshall
Environmental Policy Formation
  edited by Dean E. Mann
Environmental Policy Implementation
  edited by Dean E. Mann
The Analysis of Judicial Reform
  edited by Philip L. Dubois
The Politics of Judicial Reform
  edited by Philip L. Dubois
Critical Issues in Health Policy
  edited by Ralph Straetz, Marvin Lieberman, and Alice Sardell

Contents

Foreword

This book presents the current thinking and status of research on key issues of national importance in the health- and medical-care sector. Policy analysts view the world from a somewhat different vantage point than do basic or applied researchers. They take the findings from the two latter groups and add the dimensions of social science, political science, and economics to their analyses. This technique permits the reasoned estimation of desirability, acceptability, and feasibility of the contemplated policy.

This book provides a compendium of the thoughts of several policy analysts, including perspectives on the past as well as on current pressing issues that require consideration. The authors have recommended goals, ideas, and, where possible, short-term solutions to rather complex multifaceted issues that affect and complement the health- and medical-care-delivery systems. These authors have provided a wealth of information from their direct observation of the health sector in the United States and abroad that they have augmented with supporting literature. They have incorporated their perceptions and interpretations of these bits of information into a broad analytical framework. They conclude with their impressions or diagnoses and recommendations that appear as therapeutic measures to treat the ailing health-care sector. These are provided for consideration by the decision makers and policymakers.

These chapters are exceptionally stimulating, and I am delighted that this expanded version of a Policy Studies Organization symposium provides a wider audience for review and debate of the critical issues. We at the National Center for Health Services Research are pleased that we were able to play a part in support of this effort. It complements our research agenda, which includes many of the key issues that are the subject and concern of leading health-policy analysts, as evidenced by the writings of the panel of experts presented in this document.

Gerald Rosenthal, Ph.D.
Director
National Center for Health Services Research
Office of Health Research, Statistics, and
Technology, DHHS

Preface and Acknowledgments

Readers of the *Policy Studies Journal* should be familiar with the divergencies in goals and methods employed by policy analysts in every substantive area. This book, and indeed any work in health policy, is no exception. The authors share an interest in viewing the role of government in health care in a dynamic way— the essence of health-policy analysis. This common interest, however, does not mask the sharp differences in approach that reflect the variety of disciplinary and theoretical orientations the contributors bring to their subjects. The editors sought chapters that explore different facets of health policy from different ideological perspectives, varying from those who look to market solutions for problems in health care to those who apply a radical analysis from the "left."

This book reflects the editors' judgment on the important issues and arenas in health for policy analysis. The introductory section contains two chapters that review various approaches to health-policy analysis and explore problems of definition. The next four sections deal in turn with the questions of change and the health system, planning and regulation, financing, and issues of comparative health care.

Acknowledgments

The Policy Studies Organization gratefully thanks the U.S. Department of Health and Human Services for its financial aid to the symposium on which this book is based. Thanks are particularly owed to Gerald Rosenthal of the National Center for Health Services Research. However, no one other than the individual authors is responsible for the ideas advocated here.

Part I
Introduction

1

Health-Policy Analysis: Some Reflections on the State of the Art

David Falcone

Academics frequently are chided for their seeming preoccupation with definitions but, as has been remarked of admen and executioners, somebody has to do it. Moreover, as will be pointed out in the ensuing discussion, definitional boundaries often have significant impacts, which is part of the reason they tend to provoke heated debate. The discussion sets forth some major definitional *issues* in delimiting the field of health-policy analysis. The emphasis on issues reflects the fact that definitions will not be attempted. The field is multifaceted and, partly because it is interdisciplinary, dynamic, and relatively new, it has not undergone much of the self-examination it will have to endure as it matures. This chapter is part of the initial stirrings of that effort and purports merely to convey a glimpse of the landscape. (When it is over, the reader might suggest that a look through a kaleidoscope would have been a more apt metaphor.)

The first section deals with health; health policy; and health-services research, planning, and administration. Following this, a presupposition of the issue of the *Policies Study Journal* on which this book is based—that is, that there is validity (utility) in recognizing health-policy analysis as a field—is treated as a working hypothesis. In so doing, questions are raised about the distinctiveness of health as a policy area. Finally, the state of the art of health-policy analysis is briefly reviewed.

Health Policy

Several types of policy directly affect or seek to affect health. Those that come readily to mind are primarily legislative but also judicial and public administrative decisions dealing with: the rates of production, geographic and specialty distribution of health manpower; health-care financing; assurance of the quality of health personnel, institutions, and services; occupational safety and environmental protection; and attempts to limit consumption of presumably destructive substances such as alcohol, tobacco, and synthetic carcinogens. In some instances, the indirect effects on health of housing, income maintenance, or other welfare policies may be even more consequential than the direct effects of policies that patently deal with health. Nevertheless, it is useful to limit the conception of health policy to the conventional notion of public decisions that seek primarily to affect health or principal actors—professional and institutional—in their roles in the health arena. Indeed, employing this restriction allows one to make statements such as the previous one positing that some other policies may ultimately have a more telling impact on health than more strictly health policies, or that there is a need for integrating different policy areas (health and welfare are perhaps those most frequently cited.)[1]

Health and Health Care

If health-policy analysis is bounded by its subject matter, then the question arises as to what is meant by health and health care. That there is no dearth of literature on this topic is understandable in light of the fact that the prevalent societal conception of health at any given time obviously has profound consequences for policy. For the Greeks, health was a state of harmony, and some commentators such as Henry Sigerist think that "this is still the best general explanation we have."[2] To some extent this conception is beginning to be institutionalized in the form of the holistic-health movement.

A less romantic view is that health simply is freedom from disease. In either conception, however, as David Banta has put it, "health care could become a tyranny" if defined too broadly, particularly in the case of mental illness and chronic disease (for example, in some ways aging at a certain point could be viewed as an illness).[3] Currently the most widely cited definition of health, that posited by the World Health Organization, if implemented, might invite the tyranny that concerns Banta. According to this definition, health is a "state of complete physical, mental and social well-being and not merely the absence of disease or infirmity."[4] When one takes into consideration the perceptual (for example, what is "pain") and social (for example, what is "disability") factors involved in the determination of what constitutes health and disease, there is almost no limit to the scope of health care.

A new issue has been raised by the quantification of health-status indices,[5] incorporating social as well as biological factors, which would seem to require some decision about composite cut-off points to designate a threshold of health. The activism of one's orientation then would determine where one would make the cut.

Related to the activism-passivism continuum on which health, and thus health care, can be conceived is the differentiation between personal-health and public-health services. This distinction is more marked in the United States than in other countries, but it is ubiquitous. Briefly, the public-health perspective envisions health in terms of populations or groups whereas, in the extreme, personal-health services are delivered in a mythically unique doctor (or presumably some other health professional) to patient relationship.[6] This distinction is shaded in particular instances (for example, family practitioners supposedly view their patients in the context of their families and communities, and the public-health service does deliver health care to individuals), but it exists in reality and motivates profound differences in attitudes toward policy. For example, the American Public Health Association has traditionally supported comprehensive universal and publically administered national-health-insurance programs in opposition to representatives of the personal-health-care sector such as the American Medical Association and, to a lesser extent, the American Hospital Association.

Generally speaking, those with a public-health orientation also tend to take a relatively more active stance on sumptuary policies such as those relating to tobacco and alcohol. With some oversimplification, one could say that when the inevitable clashes between individual liberty and perceived public good occur, the public-health persuasion tends to emphasize the latter. Health-policy analysis subsumes both these schools of thought.

Overlapping to some extent the public-personal health dichotomy is another continuum on which conceptions of health care can be arrayed according to the degree to which health is recognized as a right. Until recently, the dominant view was that health was a public good; that is, that society at large received a collective benefit from the provision of a minimal level of aggregate health, that it was in each *individual's* best interest for government to *impose* a measure of health care. The most clearly justifiable policies under this rubric were those dealing with sanitation and communicable disease, to which later were added programs targeted at the disabled children and mothers. With the demise of classic liberalism and the ascendance of a reform liberalism holding that rights could be derived as well as natural, health increasingly was recognized as a right, the spread of this view was made possible by advances in the efficacy of medical care. The semingly abated escalation of such advances and increasingly constrained resources have probably subdued the enthusiasm of some proponents of the notion that health care is a right.

Health and health care obviously are portmanteau terms, as illustrated by the foregoing catalog of conceptions. They all are within the ambit of health-policy analysis and often underly scholarly and public debate, for example, whether the "health" care of the elderly is becoming "overmedicalized."

Policy

The problem of deriving a useful definition of health-policy analysis is further complicated by the problem of defining policy. The problem is imposing not because of the scarcity of meanings with some currency but the lack of commonly accepted conceptions. If they have an underlying dimension, it would be that of an *orientation* that forms the basis for decision rules, whether the decisions are what Amatai Etzioni has called "bit" or "contextuating." [7] In this view, a given policy may virtually preordain that all legislative, bureaucratic, judicial, and administrative actions would be regarded as of the "bit" variety, that is, serially incremental but part of a shifting policy context. The evolution of the welfare state—at least up until the mid-70s—is an example of this pattern. The policy toward societal (via government) responsibility for the equality of opportunity and maintenance of a minimally acceptable standard of living has been loosely formulated so as not to collide with the shibboleths of classic liberalism. Therefore, the actions (or outputs) that have occurred under its aegis such as the Maternal and Child Health/Crippled Children Services Program under the Social Security Act, the Kerr-Mills federal-state conditional granting program to provide care for the elderly poor, the Comprehensive Health Planning Program, Regional Medical Program, Medicare, and Medicaid have been targeted to specific beneficiaries or problem areas as resources have permitted and groups have "demanded."

When we think of policy as an orientation, however, we usually think of a "contextuating" government action; viz., one that explicitly initiates a new government strategy for attacking a problem and sets the stage for further predictable actions. The Social Security Act is a prime example, although even it can be viewed as a pragmatic, episodic response to a perceived crisis. The distinction between contextuating and bit policy is drawn here not so much to set forth a rudimentary typology as to indicate that what we really are distinguishing are explicit and implicit policies. There has been little in the way of distinctively contextuating policy dealing with health, although some have so regarded the 1949 Hospital Survey and Construction (Hill-Burton) Act since it marked the legitimacy of at least a measure of government-induced health planning, and medicare since it was a health as opposed to welfare (that is, it is not means tested) program.

For this reason, there is a reigning claim that we have no national health policy. (Related to this is the claim that we have no health system but rather a collage of modes of health-services delivery.) In the perspective suggested in the foregoing discussion, this claim turns into one that holds that the financing and organization of health care is not yet a government priority, that the United States has not decided to launch an articulated, coordinated movement toward the assumption of social responsibility for health and the attempt to make health services universally available and accessible.

Health-Services Research, Planning, and Administration

Health-policy analysis may or may not fall under the general heading of health-services research depending on the expansiveness of one's conception of the latter term. But health-services research, perhaps more than any other pursuit, lays the groundwork for health-policy analysis. Health-services research has been defined as:

concerned with problems in the organization, staffing, financing, utilization, and evaluation of health services. This is in contrast to biomedical research which is oriented to the etiology, diagnosis and treatment of disease. Health services research subsumes both medical care and patient care research. It could well be termed "socio-medical" research.[8]

The field is by now advanced enough to be recognized by the acronym HSR, and an entire volume[9] and other literature have been devoted to its meaning. This paper clearly cannot do justice to the field. However, some of the major subissues involved in its development can be cursorily identified[10]: that is, whether HSR should be "applied" or "basic," discipline rewarding or policy oriented, "in" health (with the health field as the principal focus) or "of" health (with disciplinary exploitation of topics in the health area as a primary motivating factor). These largely coincident distinctions can be consequential for research funding (applied research, by and large, is more attractive to dollars). However, whether research is applied is fundamentally an empirical question and thus must, a priori, pose an impressive challenge to a grantor to divine the motives of the researcher. Otherwise, one does not know whether research was basic or applied until its consequences have been evaluated.

One aspect of the basic-applied distinction that surfaces in policy studies is in the form of policy advocacy versus analysis.[11] Perhaps this is a more frank and useful dichotomy than that used in HSR because it self-consciously recognizes motives as its basis: Basic becomes "objective" (or, at least, intersubjective) in orientation; applied can be termed "adversarial" or *explicitly* value laden.

HSR and health-policy analysis dovetail in their focus; possibly the distinguishing trait of the latter is a more macroscopic and government-program-centered purview. And here it should be reaffirmed that if policy is to have any meaning, it must be reserved to government (or, to invoke a term commonly used in the health field to denote private agencies with some government sanctioning power, "subgovernmental") decisions.

With regard to the distinguishing features of health-policy analysis, planning and administration, John Kralewski, as chairman of the Task Force (of the Accrediting Commission for Graduate Education in Health Services Administration) on Specialized Accreditation for Policy Analysis, Planning and Administration Programs, has attempted to, as he wisely puts it, place some signposts to delimit the boundaries of each field.[12] What emerges from his efforts is a vision of boundaries that are hazy but discernible, with health administration occupying the acreage characterized by management skills and an institutional focus, planning sharing this turf but emphasizing different skills and outlooks (less institutionally defensive, for example), and policy analysis nomadically covering these areas but moving toward a separate area sparsely populated by traditional academic disciplines and increasingly inhabited by a new breed of hybrid health administration (or public health), that is, discipline-educated researcher. Kralewski's work is in the initial stages; it is cited here as representative of an effort, grounded in pragmatic considerations, to delimit fields of education that reflect areas of inquiry and practice. His preliminary writing suggests that the most problematic field to isolate may be health-policy analysis.

Health-Policy Analysis as an Area Study

Having attempted to examine some of the issues involved in a definition of health policy, the question arises as to whether it is valid to classify a field of inquiry by its substantive target—the institutions and principal actors involved—as opposed as to some other basis such as its effects on the distribution or allocation of resources. The question obviously has a logical dimension, but it also has pragmatic and pedagogical overtones.

One way of addressing this dilemma is to inquire as to distinctive features of the health system as an object of government action and then decide whether these characteristics warrant constituting a subheading of policy study—eschewing the issue of whether the volume of literature and the sheer numbers of people engaged in health-policy analysis requires recognizing the field as a pursuit that it would be appropriate to delimit. Undertaking this endeavor, of course, amounts to treating the assumption of this volume as an hypothesis.

With regard to process variables, there obviously are institutional actors distinctive to the health field—the four health subcommittees of Congress, for example, or health agencies of the Department of Health and Human Services. There also are myriad interest groups with an overriding interest in health policy such as the American Medical Association, the American Hospital Association, the Federation of American Hospitals (representing propietary hospitals), the American Health Care Association (representing propietary nursing homes), the American Nursing Association, the National League for Nursing, and the Association of American Medical Colleges. These groups can be expected to exert influence on all major issues. However, this is a relatively trivial distinction since the same could be said for any policy area. In fact, focusing health-policy analysis on characteristics of such institutions because they are putatively health-policy centered might obscure generalizations about administrative behavior. In short, health-policy studies are open to the same criticisms as those leveled against area studies in comparative politics.

Area studies have been defended in this regard on the basis of the special knowledge that accrues from an intensive interdisciplinary understanding of a county or region. The same grounds could be used to justify health-policy analysis if a lietmotiv for health policy can be demonstrated. One may be found in that until recently health policy has been unique in defying the liberal democratic tradition that has been the mainstream of development for other types of policy. The specific form this has taken has been the appropriation of the authority of the state to sanction medical, professional dominance and autonomy. It is true that the presence of disproportionate power relations characterizes political struggles in all policy areas. Nevertheless, the degree to which this is the case in the health field and the fact that it has been explicit marks a deviation from the norm. Granted this is a distinctive trait, does it justify a policy-area approach? Not logically since, in fact, it is a transarea perspective that highlights it. However, taking a transarea policy approach toward health without the intensified focus might not let us see that what we have termed professional dominance is a significant aberration that touches the roots of American democracy.

In a functionalist vein, we would expect professional dominance to wane since it is anomalous and, indeed, it shows signs of doing so. It seems that the United States is attempting to inject into the system a dram of classical liberal democratic spirit (which has resurged in other policy areas, displacing reform liberalism, in the past few years) via regulations such as certificate of need and peer and utilization review.

If one accepts that the primary reason for segregating health-policy analysis is the marked deviance of health policy with respect to the balance of power of interested parties and, relatedly, the relatively low salience of health issues for the general public, then it would seem that this facet of the field would be the most exploited by research. This may be true of medical sociology, but except for a few outstanding studies (such as Robert Alford's *Health Care Politics*, which won the Woodrow Wilson award in 1976),[13] political scientists and economists have ignored this phenomenon and devoted their attention to aspects of the political process in which a health focus could be viewed as almost incidental.

One way to categorize the body of health-policy analysis that permits some contrasts to be drawn with other policy-area studies and points up needed research is according to whether the relationships stressed (if this is done with any measure of explicitness) are input-process, process-output, output-outcome, or whether the systems approach is employed wherein input-process-output-outcome linkages (or the first two of them) are assessed simultaneously. There are probably fewer of the latter in health policy than in education and welfare, and those studies that have been "systemic" seem to be primarily disciplinary, that is, in the policy analysis "of" health mode.

There hardly is a voluminous literature in health-policy analysis, but relative to other policy areas, with the possible exception of education, a disproportionate amount of it seems to focus on the determinants of outcomes. A substantial body of program-evaluation research has been conducted. Unfortunately, the resulting store of verifiable generalizations does not strike much optimism for those other policy areas with an, as yet, scarce amount of such research. For example, the debate noted earlier about what constitutes health clouds the definitiveness of outcome evaluation. Another example is that outcome evaluation in health shares the problems of multicollinearity that plague similar research in other areas. For example, although screening programs are thought to have been efficacious in reducing cervical-uterine cancer mortality, the disease already was declining as a linear function of time.[14] Or, since so many diseases are self-limiting or of unknown etiology, it is difficult to attribute reduction in morbidity to programs with this intention. Nevertheless, these studies have utility if only because they raise such questions, forcing implicit assumptions into the open.

Perhaps as surprising as the comparatively large amount of attention devoted to outcomes in health-policy analysis is the relative lack of process-output studies. The legislative process in health policy has been the subject of some research—for example, Ted Marmor's *Politics of Medicare*,[15] Richard Redman's *Dance of Legislation*,[16] and David Price's "Policy Making in Congressional Committees"[17]—but major pieces of legislation, or the fact that there has been a lack of them, have gone largely unexplored. And, returning to the issue discussed earlier about the distinctiveness of health policy, in the three works cited, it is not the "health" aspects of the policies that are highlighted for their roles in the legislative process but expected redistributed impact (Marmor), degree of salience and conflict (Price), and personalities and characteristics of the congressional process (Redman). Whether this is true generally of health legislation is problematic, but so far the burden of proof would seem to be on those who would argue that variables intrinsic to the health field are significant determinants of the legislative process regarding health issues.

The bureaucratic/administrative process in health policy remains a largely unchartered domain. Studies such as Judy Feder's *Medicare*,[18] which attempts to show that the implementation of this policy was affected in large part by the fact it was administered by insurance rather than health-oriented officials, are rare. There even is a paucity of descriptive literature in this area, notwithstanding the number of government publications of this nature.

The courts and health law have been more extensively studied, but again there is very little that is specific to the health field that would distinguish this literature. Possible exceptions in light of earlier discussion are those works that deal with the incongruity of professional dominance.

Health Systems Agencies (quasi-governmental in the sense that they have delegated review powers that are subject to administrative appeal and that they are expected to work with local and regional government entities) seem to have been studied more extensively—if nowhere near adequately—than the legislature or the bureaucracy for their role in health-policy determination. This may signal that their actions are more significant in the policy process or, simply, that they (and their forerunners, the Comprehensive Health Planning Agencies) are more accessible research sites. Research on HSAs has been largely concerned with the relations among state, local, and federal agencies, and board representativeness and degree of consumer participation. Therefore, the focus has been on process with, at least implicitly, a *presumed* effect on outputs and outcomes.

Inputs and processes have been the subject of considerable research, characterized generally by a more or less explicit "group" approach. Congruent with what was said earlier about the distinctiveness of certain groups to policy fields (that is, excluding the business, labor, civic action, partisan-ideological and consumer groups that can be expected to air views on any or all issues), the health-policy process has been dominated by their sentiments and interests. The policy relevance of these studies depends on one's judgment about the importance for outputs and outcomes of the group struggle. There is little doubt in the case of the health field that group interests have affected policies. But whether the effects have been determining still seems a matter of speculation.

Summary

This chapter has aired some major issues in health-policy analysis through a discussion of definitional problems and a consideration of the distinctiveness of the field. In surveying the scope of health-policy analysis, health policy has been limited to its conventional usage—that is, government decisions and actions that have the overt intention of affecting the health system—while noting the significant impact on the system that policies in other areas may have. For example, changes in laws regarding the tax treatment of nonprofit institutions would have important consequences for hospitals, the majority of which fall in this category, but if hospitals were not the chief concern of these policies, one would not label them health policies. This restriction allows for a comparison of the relative influence on health care of different policy areas.

In a brief examination of the meaning of policy, it was argued that this term usually is equated with explicit contextuating policy when, in fact, the nature of a policy may not really be apparent until the flow of decisions that issue from it has occurred. Thus it may not be entirely correct to say that the United States has no health policy; rather, it may have a health policy consonant with the vestiges of classical liberalism in our political culture.

Since health-policy analysis is not a methodological or functional but a subject-matter-oriented field, some of the protean conceptions of health and health care were explored. It was pointed out that the shape and direction of health policy is inextricable from the prevailing societal view of what constitutes health.

The closest thing to a disciplinary basis for health-policy analysis is, in fact, an interdisciplinary amalgam called health-services research. In identifying

HSR, the chapter reviewed a preliminary effort to differentiate health-policy analysis, planning, and administration as fields of education, inquiry, and practice.

Finally, the literature in health-policy analysis was assessed in light of its relative attention to input-process, process-output, and output-outcome linkages. Hopefully somewhat short of breast beating, the question was raised as to whether a subject-matter focus such as health is an appropriate subclassification of policy analysis. It was contended that the resolution of this issue rests on whether health policy is distinctive with respect to the processes involved in its formulation and that this has not been demonstrated by the research to date. In fact, a transarea policy focus is needed to settle this question.

Notes

1. See, for example, Gerben DeJong, "Interfacing National Health Insurance and Income Maintenance: Why Health and Welfare Reform Go Together," *Journal of Health Politics, Policy and Law* 1 (Winter 1977):405-432.

2. *Medicine and Human Welfare* (College Park, Md.: McGrath, 1970), p. 46, cited in David Banta, "What is Health Care?" in *Health Care Delivery in the United States,* ed. Steven Jonas (New York: Springer), p. 14.

3. Banta, "What is Health Care?", p. 21.

4. World Health Organization, "The Constitution of the World Health Organization," *WHO Chronicle* 1 (1944).

5. See W. Balinksy and R. Berger, "A Review of Research on General Health Status Indices," *Medical Care* 13 (1975).

6. The distinction is highlighted in an exchange in the *Journal of Health Politics, Policy and Law* 2 (Spring 1977): Sagar Jain, "Whither Education in Public Health?" and Cecil Sheps, "Reply to Jain."

7. "Mixed Scanning: A 'Third' Approach to Decision-Making," *Public Administration Review* 27 (December 1967):385-92.

8. E. Evelyn Flook and Paul Sanazaro, "Health Services Research: Origins and Milestones," in *Health Services Research and R&D in Perspective,* eds. Flook and Sanazaro (Ann Arbor, Mich.: Health Administration Press, 1973), p. 1.

9. Ibid.

10. For amplification of these issues, see Robert Eichorn and Thomas Bice, "Academic Disciplines and Health Services Research," in *Health Services Research,* eds. E. Evelyn Flook and Paul Sanazaro, pp. 136-149.

11. See, for example, Thomas Dye, *Understanding Public Policy*, 3rd ed. (Englewood Cliffs, N.J.: Prentice-Hall, 1978), chap. 1.

12. "The Health Administration Domain." Paper delivered at the 1980

meeting of the Association of Univeristy Programs in Health Administration, Washington, D.C., May 10.

13. (Chicago: University of Chicago Press, 1975).

14. U.S. National Center for Health Statistics, "Age Adjusted Cancer Death Rates for Selected Sites, 1930-1975."

15. (Chicago: Aldine, 1973).

16. (New York: Simon and Schuster, 1973).

17. *American Political Science Review* 72 (June 1978):548-574.

18. (Lexington, Mass.: D.C. Heath, 1977).

2 Paradigms in the Study of Health Policy

Elianne Riska

Contemporary literature on the American health system virtually unanimously agrees that the system is facing a crisis. One can, however, distinguish four different interpretations of this crisis and its causes: an individual-deficiency, economic, organizational, and Marxist perspective. This essay will critically examine the four different interpretative frameworks as "diagnostic paradigms" (Warren 1971). *Diagnostic paradigm* in this discussion means a way of concep-tualizing a problem and what strategies will be used to deal with the problem. It is contended that such paradigms can easily be identified in most reform proposals presented to alleviate problems in American health care.

The Individual-Deficiency Perspective

A number of observers have argued that current problems in the American health system originate in people's value systems and concomitant behavioral expressions. Such behavior has been seen as explaining why health care has come to cost more, that is, because of the underutilization of preventive care or the improper use of sources of acute medical care. Although originally the lack of "rational" medical behavior was mainly attributed to the poor, more recently observers have begun to include the rest of the population as well.

How the poor look after their health has been criticized for two opposing reasons: Some propose that the poor *under*utilize health care and that is the big problem whereas others deplore that the poor *over*utilize medical care. Those who hold that the poor underutilize medical care have explained this behavior by referring to the alienation of the poor, or to a special value system held among them (see, for example, Moody and Gray 1972; Nall and Spielberg 1967; Hoppe and Heller 1975). The basic idea is that the poor are generally estranged from the mainstream of middle-class American society: the poor are alienated and apathetic toward any involvement in society, and their families are highly disorganized. This social environment has created a world view or a subculture of the poor that has left them unable to cope with requirements—from achieve-ment to bureaucracy—of the middle-class society (see Harrington 1962).

The proponents of such a sociocultural view suggest that underutilization of medical care by the poor is related to their way of life; and as Goering and Coe (1970, pp. 309-310) have suggested, "underutilization then becomes the direct result of the culture and values of the poor and presumably little or nothing can be done to improve health conditions for the poor without a change in these values." This perspective adopts what Warren (1971) has called an "individual-deficiency" model in its diagnosis of the underlying sources of the problems. Such a model suggests that it is the individual's value system that is at fault rather than the social system.

In contrast, others have suggested that the poor actually overuse health services—they are forever "doctoring." The argument here derives from Shuval's contention about the two functions of medical practice (Shuval 1970). The manifest function of medical practice is to cure illness, but another function is latent: the using of medical care as a way of channeling unmet personal, emotional needs. The alleged overuse of medical care by the poor in the United States has been examined in the light of this latent function, a function Shuval has defined as "catharsis." In a study of female welfare recipients, for example, Cole and Lejeune (1972) suggest that overutilization of medical care by the poor women was an attempt to adopt a sick role—a more acceptable form of deviance in the American society than poverty.

Those who propose the "underutilization" interpretation and those who advocate the "overutilization" interpretation base their interpretations on similar underlying assumptions. Both assume that there exists a "normal" load of medical problems that patients can be expected to present. They also implicitly advance a normative picture of what a "normal" healthy person is like. But the criteria used for a definition of such normal behavior are biased toward presenting white, male, middle-class behavior as the rational behavior. [This kind of description of "normal" behavior has a long-standing tradition in American social sciences. A classical essay on this topic is C. Wright Mills' (1943) examination of the biased view portrayed by social scientists in textbooks in the field of social disorganization.]

Yet it is not only the values of the *poor* that have been viewed as preventing rational medical behavior. Lately critics have also argued that *everybody* has taken to overutilizing medical care because of the "overmedicalization" of society. The most radical proponents of this view (Illich 1976; Carlson 1975) have argued that advancements in scientific medicine have created major threats to the health of the general public. The American population, and the middle class in particular because of its ability to consume, has succumbed to the imperialism of the medical profession. Since the population has lost its ability to take care of itself and since the medical ideology indoctrinates people to consume medical care uncritically, a generation of "overutilizers" has been born.

The negative view of the contributions of medicine to improvements in health has led to an increased attention to environmental and behavioral influences on the health status of the general population (for example, McKeown 1971, 1976). Although one would have assumed that such a view should have resulted in a revitalized interest in public health and social policy as major instruments in promoting health, the American debate has taken a different direction. The solution to major health problems has been presented as a restoration of self-care (Illich 1976; Knowles 1977). As Knowles (1977, p. 59), a notable promoter of such an approach, has suggested: "I believe the idea of a 'right' to health should be replaced by the idea of an individual moral obligation to preserve one's own health—a public duty if you will." It is Knowles's (1977: p. 61) contention that a control of the present major health problems in the United States depends directly on modification of the individual's behavior and habits of living. This means that unhealthy behavior related to affluent lifestyles or so-called self-abuse—overeating, smoking, drinking, sedentary living—should be modified to conform to an ideal of healthy behavior.

The endeavors for self-care, generally promoted and conducted by health professionals, have ranged from child-birthing classes, hypertension clinics, to a rejuvenated interest in instruction in cross-country skiing and jogging. It is argued that these measures will allow the individual not only to take care of his or her own health care but also to more rationally approach the health-care system.

Yet as a number of critics (Crawford 1977; Berliner and Salmon 1979; Kronenfeld 1979) have observed, the movement for self-care in the 1970s does not represent a "new" approach, for all the sudden upsurge of such activities. Instead, it not only expresses but also confirms a long-standing emphasis on individualism, privatism, and self-reliance in American society. In this sense, the self-care movement interprets problems as personal ones and fails to recognize the social framework that produced the broader social problem and the individual trouble. In short, the self-care approach promotes an individual-deficiency model in its diagnosis of the underlying sources of problems.

In conclusion, the individual-deficiency model on problems in American health care portrays not only users of health services as mainly responsible for the troubles but blames, in particular, the values and life styles of the individual for the problem. As observed above, an interesting shift has occurred in the focus of this view. In the 1960s, the values of the poor were held primarily responsible for problems in health care, and policy measures were directed toward eradicating these "bad values." In the 1970s, by contrast, there has been little concern about the health of the poor. Instead, it is assumed that *everybody* has succumbed to an unhealthy life style as part of living in an affluent society. But both versions of this diagnostic paradigm have proposed the same policy solution: a modification of the individual's values and life styles. This diagnosis carries a victim-blaming imputation that leads its proponents to advocate individualized solutions rather than health- or social-policy measures promoting collective solutions.

The Economic Perspective

For a number of observers of the health-care scene, the crisis is in essence a "chronic inflation of expenditures" largely caused by price inflation, product change, and increased utilization (Rice and Wilson 1976, p. 151). A review of the proportion of the gross national product (GNP) spent on health-care expenditures shows that there has been a drastic increase during the past three decades. For example, 4.5 percent of the GNP was spent on health care in 1950, 5.2 percent in 1960, 7.2 percent in 1970, and 8.8 percent in 1977. During the same time the per-capita expenditures for health care rose from $78.35 in 1950 to $333.57 in 1960, and were estimated at $736.92 in 1977. From 1974 to 1976 alone, the increase in health-care expenditures was estimated at 31 percent while the GNP increased by 18 percent (Gibson and Mueller 1977; Gibson and Fisher 1978).

But the question is, Why have the preceding economic figures become a public concern, and how does an economic perspective explain the "crisis" in the health-care sector? That is, how does an economic perspective conceptualize the problem, and what kind of intervention strategies to alleviate or possibly eliminate the crisis are most likely to be adopted.

One of the major concerns of the economists is the current character of the decision making about the allocation of resources in the medical market. The argument has been that the current health system does not lend itself to a "sound" working of the market forces and that the presence of problems within existing arrangements of health care indicates imbalances in the market system. But a review of the writings of economists on the health-care crisis suggests two different points of views: those who search for causes and solutions within a free-market model and those who ask for increased public control and regulation. The conservative economists view the struggle between numerous interest groups in the medical-care field not only as inevitable but also as necessary for the achievement of an optimum quality and quantity of medical care. According to this view a restoration of an unrestrained medical-market system would provide a solution to problems in American health care. For example, Friedman (1962, p. 262) argues that pluralism and competition among agencies, programs, institutions, and health professionals are necessary ingredients of a sound operation of a health system because "they guarantee diversity by maintaining competition between alternative modes of providing health care."

The liberal representatives, on the other hand, are not as rigidly opposed to coordination, planning of the allocation and use of health care resources, and to government involvement in general as are the conservative economists. But like the conservative economists, the liberal economists view the major problem as the "faulty incentive structure" that has been allowed to emerge since third parties have come to be involved in reimbursement for medical care. The present incentive structure, both conservative and liberal economists argue, has no built-in mechanisms for self-regulation—what has been called "economizing behavior"—either on the part of the consumer or the provider of medical care. In other words, increased reimbursement by third parties has made both consumers and providers insensitive to cost containment. Hence both the consumer and the provider are likely to opt for the use of high-cost care even when this care might do little to improve the patient's health.

As already observed, the intervention strategy to these problems proposed by the conservative economists consists of a restoration of the self-regulation of the economic market by changing the incentive structure, a measure most liberal economists are likely to support. The liberal economists do not, however, envision a balanced medical market emerging without the benign involvement of the government. As Victor Fuchs (1974), an economist with a liberal stance on health-policy issues, has noted that society has to make a choice about what kind of health-care system it wants. Such a choice would set cost-contained goals for our health needs, and such a floor would then enable planners and economists to organize a cost-effective health system. But to the more radical economists, the correct strategy would entail a total removal of health care from the economic market and the installation of it as a public utility. This strategy asks for public ownership and control of health facilities and resources, a strategy that has not yet been presented in any of the national-health-insurance proposals. The most radical proposal, the Kennedy-Corman Health Security bill, merely suggests a federally funded health system but leaves the issue of the ownership of health facilities unaddressed.

The Organizational Perspective

Unlike the conservative economists who have viewed competition among a multitude of providers, agencies, and programs as a positive phenomenon, those adopting an organizational approach have deplored this condition and argued that competition constitutes the major problem in the American health system. They believe that rampant uncoordination is the inevitable outcome of an historical lack of organization in the American health-delivery system. For example, Roemer et al. (1975, p. 2), who posit an organizational approach, view the problem as "a crisis in part related to our national health policy, described as lacking coordination, often lacking rationality, and frequently having glaring short-comings of performance." Furthermore, fragmentation of health services is, according to this view, one of the major problems.

Those presenting an organizational perspective on the nation's health-care crisis suggest as an intervention strategy organizational reform by means of centralized public regulation and planning. This reform strategy has been advocated in recent health legislation, for example, the National Health Planning and Resource Development Act of 1974 (PL 93-641), which created a structure of around 200 planning councils, the Health Systems Agencies (HSAs) (see, for example, Klarman, 1978; Rosenfeld and Rosenfeld, 1975). It is too early to judge whether these agencies have fulfilled the expectations and objectives originally given the refurbished versions of the previous Comprehensive Health Planning Agencies (CHPs) of 1967.

Perhaps a more interesting question, at least from a sociological point of view, is why these agencies have been accepted at all as regulatory agencies in a predominantly voluntary health-care system enormously resistant to change. One plausible explanation is that organizational reform has been viewed as an essentially apolitical and technical measure (see, for example, Warren 1971). In other words, it has been believed to be carried on by experts who mainly have addressed the issue of efficiency of organizational performance rather than any political dimensions of the health-care "crisis."

In short, the organizational perspective conceptualizes the main problem as the disorganization of medical care. Its proponents do not relate the problems in the health sector to principles guiding the larger society. Instead, they accept the underlying structure of society as essentially sound and suggest organizational reforms. Such an intervention strategy is assumed to improve the organizational performance of the health-care system, a circumstance that would result in reduced costs and increased access to medical care as well.

The Marxist Perspective

In contrast to the conservative economists who see unrestricted capitalism as a solution to all problems in the American health system, the advocates of a Marxist perspective view the capitalist economy itself as the source of all problems in the health sector. Recently an increasing number of authors have analyzed the problems of the American health system within the framework of this perspective (for example, Ehrenreich and Ehrenreich 1970; Waitzkin and Waterman 1974; Bodenheimer 1973; Krause 1977; Navarro 1975, 1976, 1977). The promoters of the Marxist perspective argue that the health sector reflects the lack of control over resources and wealth that we find in the society at large. In this way, the American health sector merely mirrors the class hierarchy and distribution of power of a capitalist society. But medicine has a special function in a capitalist society: It reproduces and legitimates the capitalist system (Waitzkin and Waterman 1974; Navarro 1977). The ideology of medicine complements the ideology of capitalism and medicine can, in this way, be used as a tool to depoliticize conflicts or injustices growing out of the unequal distribution of wealth, resources, and power in society because the effects of these injustices can be reduced to individual troubles.

In contrast to the three other perspectives that take the existing society as a given, the Marxist perspective demands a radical transformation of the existing society before improvements in the health sector can be looked for. Such a transformation entails a redistribution of wealth and of control over resources in the capitalist society, a society that generates the kind of injustices experienced by the poorer not only in the political and economic arena but in the health sector as well.

The way in which the problems in the health sector are conceptualized by the Marxist advocates leads them not to offer any solutions at all. It is unrealistic to assume that wealth and income in the United States will be radically redistributed within the foreseeable future. Meanwhile, some reforms, like public support of preventive medicine, maternal and child care, could be instituted, measures that would alleviate the most marked injustices in health status between the poorer and the richer. But the writings of the proponents of the Marxist perspective are devoid of pragmatic suggestions about what kind of incremental policies could be accepted and supported. Thus although this perspective offers a clear diagnosis of the problems in the health sector, it cannot suggest pragmatic intervention strategies for those who develop health policy. Nor has it provided us with a model of how an alternative health system would be designed and administered.

Conclusion

This chapter has examined four paradigms that illustrate the sources of the major problems in American health care. These paradigms are ideal types. When we study specific health-reform proposals, we find that they often will share many characteristics of different paradigms.

References

Bodenheimer, Thomas S. 1973. "Health Care in the United States: Who Pays." *International Journal of Health Services* 3:467-474.

Berliner, Howard S., and Salmon, J. Warren. 1979. "The Holistic Health Movement and Scientific Medicine: The Naked and the Dead." *Socialistic Review* 9:31-52.

Carlson, Rick J. 1975. *The End of Medicine.* New York: Wiley.

Cole, Stephen, and Lejeune, Robert. 1972. "Illness and the Legitimation of Failure." *American Sociological Review* 37:347-356.

Crawford, Robert. 1977. "You Are Dangerous to Your Health: The Ideology and Politics of Victim Blaming." *International Journal of Health Services* 7:663-679.

Ehrenreich, Barbara, and Ehrenreich, John. 1970. *The American Health Empire.* New York: Random House.

Friedman, Milton. 1962. *Capitalism and Freedom.* Chicago: University of Chicago Press.

Fuchs, Victor. 1974. *Who Shall Live?* New York: Basic Books.

Gibson, Robert J., and Mueller, Marjorie Smith. 1977. "National Health Expenditures, Fiscal Year 1976." *Social Security Bulletin* 40:3-22.

Gibson, Robert M., and Fisher, Charles R. 1978. *"National Health Expenditures, Fiscal Year 1977." Social Security Bulletin* 41:3-20.

Goering, John M., and Coe, Rodney M. 1970. "Cultural Versus Situational Explanations of the Medical Behavior of the Poor." *Social Science Quarterly* 51:309-319.

Harrington, Michael. 1962. *The Other America: Poverty in the United States.* New York: MacMillan.

Hoppe, Sue K., and Heller, Peter L. 1975. "Alienation, Familialism and Utilization of Health Services by Mexican Americans." *Journal of Health and Social Behavior* 16:304-315.

Illich, Ivan. 1976. *Medical Nemesis.* New York: Pantheon Books.

Klarman, Herbert E. 1978. "Health Planning: Progress, Prospects, and Issues." *Milbank Memorial Fund Quarterly/Health and Society* 56:78-112.

Knowles, John. 1977. "The Responsibility of the Individual." In *Doing Better and Feeling Worse: Health in the United States.* New York: Norton, pp. 57-80.

Kronenfeld, Jennie J. 1979. "Self Care as a Panacea for the Ills of the Health Care System: An Assessment." *Social Science and Medicine* 13A:263-267.

Krause, Elliott A. 1977. *Power & Illness: The Political Sociology of Health and Medical Care.* New York: Elsevier.

McKeown, Thomas. 1971. "A Historical Appraisal of the Medical Task." In Gordon McLachlan and Thomas McKeown, eds., *Medical History and Medical Care.* London: Oxford University Press, pp. 25-50.

———. 1976. *The Role of Medicine: Dream, Mirage, or Nemesis?* London: The Nuffield Provincial Hospitals Trust.

Mills, C. Wright. 1943. "The Professional Ideology of Social Pathologists." *American Journal of Sociology* 44:165-180.

Moody, Phillip, and Gray, Robert M. 1972. "Social Class, Social Integration and the Use of Preventive Health Services." In E.G. Jaco, ed., *Patients, Physicians and Illness*, 2nd ed. New York: Free Press, pp. 240-251.

Nall, Frank C., II, and Spielberg, Joseph. 1967. "Social and Cultural Factors in the Responses of Mexican Americans to Medical Treatment." *Journal of Health and Social Behavior* 8:299-309.

Navarro, Vicente. 1975. "The Political Economy of Medical Care: An Explanation of the Composition, Nature and Functions of the Present Health Sector in the United States." *International Journal of Health Services* 5: 65-94.

_____. 1976. "The Political and Economic Determinants of Health and Health Care in Rural America." *Inquiry* 8:111-121.

_____. 1977. "Social Class, Political Power, and the State and Their Implications in Medicine." *International Journal of Health Services* 7:255-293.

Rice, Dorothy P., and Wilson, Douglas. 1976. "The American Medical Economy: Problems and Perspectives." *Journal of Health Politics, Policy and Law* 1: 151-172.

Roemer, Ruth, Kramer, Charles, and Frink, Jeanne E. 1975. *Planning Urban Health Services: From Jungle to System.* New York: Springer Publishing Company.

Rosenfeld, Leonard S., and Rosenfeld, Irene. 1975. "National Health Planning in the United States: Prospects and Portents." *International Journal of Health Services* 5:441-453.

Shuval, Judith T. 1970. *Social Functions of Medical Practice.* San Francisco: Jossey-Bass.

Waitzkin, Howard, and Waterman, Barbara. 1974. *The Exploitation of Illness in Capitalist Societies.* Indianapolis: Bobbs-Merrill.

Warren, Roland. 1971. "The Sociology of Knowledge and the Problems of the Inner Cities." *Social Science Quarterly* 52:468-485.

**Part II
Dynamics of Health Policy**

3 The Mobilization of Bias in Primary-Care Policy: The Case of Neighborhood Health Centers

Alice Sardell

Introduction

The dominant perspective in American political science during the 1950s and well into the 1960s was optimism about the American policy process. It was assumed that this process included moderate change in response to emergent social needs.[1] In *Politics, Economics and Welfare*, a book first published in 1953,[2] Robert A. Dahl and Charles E. Lindbloom describe policy change as planned by an elite of "rational" men who calculate and then act, using strategies from "incrementalism to calculated risk-taking."[3] The 1976 preface to the latest edition of their book reflects the events within both the American polity and the field of political science in the intervening twenty-three years. The questions are different now. They are no longer about the way in which a policymaker can best manage change, but rather, whether (and possibly how) "reform" can take place at all.[4] In the words of Dahl and Lindblom, "If societies move forward, they do so not simply because from time to time reformers mobilize their energies, but because from time to time they manage to outwit, bypass and dominate the many energies that are mobilized, often knowingly, against reform."[5]

Although there is a large body of theoretical work by critics of pluralism about the "biased" nature of the American political process,[6] there are fewer studies that attempt to examine exactly how the "mobilization of bias" operates within a specific policy area to deflect attempts at change.[7] The focus of this chapter is on the nature of power relationships within the primary-care sector of American health policy over time and the operation of the "mobilization of bias" in maintaining those relationships.

The definition of "primary care" has been the subject of some debate,[8] but it will be defined here as health services that are provided on an ambulatory or outpatient basis, and "basic or general health care which emphasizes the point when the *patient* first seeks assistance from the medical care system and the care of the simpler and more common *illnesses*."[9]

In this chapter, the major elements of the "mobilization of bias" in U.S. primary-care policy will first be briefly discussed. It will then be argued that neighborhood health centers, comprehensive health-care programs funded by the federal government beginning in 1965, were a potential challenge to the structural arrangements maintained by that "mobilization of bias." For this reason, the neighborhood health-center program did not initially enter the "channel of policy choices" as part of the health-policy agenda. Rather, it was considered as part of a separate agenda, that of the War on Poverty.

Before discussing primary-care policy, it is first necessary to review the concepts of non-decision making and the mobilization of bias to discuss their limitations as analytic tools, and to suggest one way in which these limitations can be overcome.

The Concepts of the Mobilization of Bias and Non-Decision Making

Bachrach and Baratz's contribution (in *Power and Poverty*[10]) to the analysis of the functioning of the American political process was made within the context of the debate over the measurement of power within local communities. Their major critique of the pluralists was that by focusing on the decision-making process alone, these analysts ignored the questions of why certain issues and not others are on the political agenda, and whether all individuals and groups have an equal chance to place issues on that agenda. By choosing to study power as it is used on "significant issues," the pluralists limited themselves to the study of only one "face of power."[11] "Power is also exercised when A devotes his energies to creating or reinforcing social and political values and institutional practices that limit the scope of the political process to public consideration of only those issues which are comparatively innocuous to A."[12] In other words, "political systems" and "subsystems" develop a "mobilization of bias,"

> a set of predominant values, beliefs, rituals and institutional procedures ("rules of the game") that operate systematically and consistently to the benefit of certain persons and groups at the expense of others. Those who benefit are placed in a preferred position to defend and promote their vested interests.[13]

Bachrach and Baratz identify the means by which a certain mobilization of bias is sustained as non-decision making. Non-decision making involves the ways in which

> demands for change in the existing allocation of benefits and privileges in the community can be suffocated before they are even voiced; or kept covert; or killed before they gain access to the relevant decision-

making area; or failing all these things, maimed or destroyed in the decision-implementing stage of the policy process.[14]

While Bachrach and Baratz's work is a major step toward conceptualizing the way that change is limited within the American policy system, there are obstacles to its use in analyzing empirical data. First, the position that Bachrach and Baratz take on the issue of how the mobilization of bias can be studied makes their general argument somewhat ambiguous. In describing the concepts of the mobilization of bias and non-decision making, they are referring to a set of rule-making processes or political institutions and an ideology ("values and beliefs") that maintain certain power arrangements within a society. Yet in describing a methodology for studying non-decision making, they seem to be saying that there are *discrete*, specific exercises of power that occur in response to specific challenges to the prevailing mobilization of bias and that these can be observed.[15] When describing or defining non-decision making, they say that "demands for change in the existing allocation of benefits . . . can be suffocated before they are even voiced. . . ."[16] If they are suffocated before they are even voiced, then how can they be observed? If the mobilization of bias is operating successfully from the perspective of dominant groups, then it will not shift in favor of new or challenging groups as Bachrach and Baratz found that it did in Baltimore.[17]

The second but related issue concerns the measurement of change. The subject of Bachrach and Baratz's case study, antipoverty policy in Baltimore and its relation to "an ideology of white supremacy,"[18] is an area in which the content of the mobilization of bias is fairly straightforward.[19] In addition, the measurement of a shift in the mobilization of bias could be approximated in terms of outcomes such as membership of blacks on antipoverty boards and the actual distribution of income. In other areas such as health policy, determining the content of the mobilization of bias itself is a far more complex issue.

One way to deal with both of these problems is to analyze the existing structural arrangements and the mobilization of bias that helps to maintain them in a specific policy area. A particular mobilization of bias can be viewed as having developed historically as a result of a series of previous events or decisions. Once the specific structural arrangements within a particular sector of the economy or society and the specific content of the mobilization of bias within that policy area have been described, it is then possible to analyze whether non-decision making has worked to maintain that existing mobilization of bias or whether a policy change has indeed occurred.

In the next section of this chapter, the mobilization of bias in primary care policy will be briefly outlined. In another work, the historical development of the primary-care sector of the U.S. health system is discussed in greater detail.[20]

The Structure of the Primary-Care Sector

The basic arrangements for the provision of primary care in the United States in the early 1960s had already taken shape by the 1920s. Personal-health services were to be provided by the private sector; in the 1920s this was the fee-for-service physician in solo practice. The hospital outpatient department would also provide primary care, but only to charity patients as determined by a means test. The use of such means tests reinforced the first element of the mobilization of bias in primary care, the dominance of the private sector of medicine.

Means tests were instituted in both hospital outpatient departments and freestanding dispensaries after a campaign by the organized medical profession against "dispensary abuse" at the end of the nineteenth century. This campaign was part of a larger effort to reduce competition for patients and thereby improve the economic position of private practitioners.[21] A means test would assure that only those individuals willing to publicly label themselves as charity patients would have an alternative to private practice as a source of medical care.

The historian Charles Rosenberg has pointed out that the concept of "dispensary abuse" had an important ideological function in terms of the direction of health policy. If "abuse" (fraud) was *not* the explanation for the fact that many people were seeking care at dispensaries, then "large numbers of worthy and hard-working Americans were indeed too poor to pay for even minimally adequate medical care."[22] In that case, the adequacy of private arrangements might be questioned. As it developed, however, the role of the public sector was limited to one that would not be competitive with private medicine.

In New York City, for example, professionals working within the Department of Health during the Progressive period attempted to expand the scope of its activities. They met with opposition from the medical community. In 1914, Health Commissioner Sigismund S. Goldwater initiated a series of policies that would involve the Health Department in the direct provision of services.[23] At a meeting of one medical group, "the Health Department was accused of virtually committing the city 'to a policy of Socialism' and its health programs were described as 'ruinous to the business of the medical practitioners of the city.' "[24]

Goldwater's tenure as commissioner was quite short, and during a period of budget tightening under the next health commissioner (1915), the city's nose and throat clinics for children were closed. This was "a step which the Public Health Committee of the New York Academy of Medicine heartily approved."[25] "As long as the department's medical inspectors merely reported thousands of physical defects among school children, the medical profession had no objection, but the opening of clinics to correct these conditions was another story."[26] In New York, as in other areas, local public-health departments offered only those services that private physicians were unable to provide or uninterested in providing.

The federal government remained largely uninvolved in the health system until the 1930s. At that time money was provided to the states to purchase medical care for the poor from the private sector and/or to support local government health services limited to specific demographic (infants) or disease (TB patients) categories.

The second element of the structure of American primary care was the clear separation of responsibility for the health of individuals from that of responsibility for the health of large populations. The first phase of the public-health movement in the latter part of the nineteenth century had been concerned with health as a product of the physical and social environment. This changed under the influence of the new science of bacteriology. The public-health movement, like medicine in general, focused on specific disease as manifest within the individual patient.[27]

A third element, and one not limited to either the primary-care sector of the health system nor to the United States, was the dominance of physicians in the process of decision making about health care.[28]

The Neighborhood Health Center as a Challenge to the Prevailing Mobilization of Bias

Neighborhood health centers (nhcs), first funded in 1965 as research and demonstration projects by the Office of Economic Opportunity's (OEO) Community Action program, were to represent a new "model" of health-services organization that would provide dignified, accessible, "comprehensive care." Health workers, including physicians, would operate in "teams," residents of the area in which the center was located would be employed in paraprofessional positions, social-service and "outreach" services were to be provided, and there was to be "community participation" in the governance of the centers. Health centers were to serve all the residents of a particular community.[29]

The neighborhood health-center model challenged the existing health-care-delivery system in several ways. First, it was to reintegrate the traditional separation between public-health and personal-health services by defining "health" broadly and providing preventive, environmental and outreach services as well as medical treatment at one facility. Second, by providing care to *all* the residents of a geographically defined community rather than to those who passed a means test for poverty or fit certain demographic or disease categories, health centers were disregarding the boundaries between public and private medicine that had previously been negotiated. Third, the neighborhood health center was a form of group practice employing salaried physicians and thus challenged the fee-for-service solo-practice model of health care advocated and defended by organized medicine. The team concept of health manpower organization challenged the traditional medical hierarchy. Finally, professional dominance was also challenged by the notion of consumer participation in decisions about health-care services.

It was precisely because the nhc model challenged the basic structure of the American health-care system that it could be considered only as part of a separate agenda, one limited to the poor. The two reformist physicians who wrote the proposal for the first neighborhood health center had originally taken their health-center plan to officials in the Public Health Service within HEW. These officials sent them to OEO,[30] an agency without established relationships to provider groups. Even so, after the decision was made that the Office of Economic Opportunity would fund some experimental centers, OEO officials reassured the American Medical Association (AMA) that health centers *"would not interfere with existing private practices of AMA constituents* whose practice usually did not extend to large numbers of medically indigent patients."[31] A program limited to the poor would not challenge the existing structural arrangements described above.[32]

Although the "health establishment" did not oppose the neighborhood health-center program, and in fact hospitals participated in it, the program did have its active opponents. At the national level, Southern politicians opposed the program, as they did the rest of the War on Poverty, because they did not wish potential political resources—such as money and jobs—to be provided to Southern blacks by the federal government. At the local level, opposition came from pharmacists in communities where the health center would include a pharmacy, from black physicians in Northern ghetto areas, and from officials of Southern public-health departments: those whose "turf" was being threatened.[33] It is significant that those who initially opposed the neighborhood health-center program were *the least powerful* of those benefiting from the existing mobilization of bias in primary-care health policy. The most powerful groups (the AMA and the hospitals) did not need to engage in interest-group politics since their interests had already been anticipated by federal policymakers.

While grants for health centers were to be made to groups and institutions in low-income areas, the program did not initially require a means test for individuals seeking health care at the centers. In 1967, however, just one year after Congress had authorized specific funding for neighborhood health centers,[34] an amendment to the OEO Act was passed that changed the eligibility criterion from residence in a center's catchment area to income below the poverty level. This amendment, sponsored by private practitioners, effectively prevented neighborhood health centers from serving a mixed-income clientele and thus expanding beyond a poverty population.[35]

The validity of examining the characteristics of a given set of structural arrangements as the first step in analyzing the operation of the mobilization of bias is shown by the fact that the most directly challenging aspect of the nhc model was the first to be undone. The 1967 OEO amendment reinstituted the means test. Federal support for a new model of health-care delivery was clearly to be only for that part of the population that was unable to purchase care from the private sector.

Conclusion: Neighborhood Health Centers and the Mobilization of Bias

In a paper on the politics of national health insurance, Richard E. Cairl and Allen W. Imershein assert that "the prevailing mobilization of bias can be examined from at least two perspectives. . . ."[36] One is the role of the federal government in relation to the provision of social services; the other is reform of the health-care-delivery system itself. The enactment of medicare was a shift in the mobilization of bias from the first perspective since the federal government was to assume a new role in the financing of health services. This, however, was to be done without any change in the organization of health care.

Cairl and Imershein also argue that in the postmedicare period "dominant structural interests" in medicine continue to be able to "restrict" discussion in health policy to financing issues.[37] The mobilization of bias is operating when such interests are able "to influence what alternatives are considered legitimate in the first place."[38] Theodore Marmor, while he does not use Bachrach and Baratz's terms, finds that his study of the passage of medicare "illustrated the capacity of the AMA to influence the agenda of discussion and to limit the alternatives policymakers could suggest."[39] Similarly, it has been argued here that the neighborhood health-center model contained several elements that challenged the existing mobilization of bias in the organization of health care and for this reason could become only part of the policy agenda under the rubric of the War on Poverty. Defined as a program to provide health services to low-income individuals, the nhc model did not threaten the existing organizational and financial arrangements within the mainstream health system.

Notes

1. The "classic" statement about the activation of "potential groups" in response to changes in the social equilibrium is, of course, found in David B. Truman, *The Government Process, Political Interests and Public Opinion* (New York: Alfred A. Knopf, 1951).

2. Robert A. Dahl and Charles E. Lindblom, *Politics, Economics and Welfare: Planning and Political Economic Systems Resolved into Basic Social Processes* (Chicago: University of Chicago Press, 1953; reprinted 1976).

3. Ibid., pp. 82-88.

4. Ibid., pp. xl-xli.

5. Ibid., p. xl.

6. For example, E.E. Schattschneider, *The Semisovereign People: A Realist's View of Democracy in America* (New York: Holt, Rinehart and Winston, 1960); Wiliam E. Connolly, ed., *The Bias of Pluralism* (New York: Atherton Press, 1969); Grant McConnell, *Private Power and American Democracy* (New York: Vintage Books, 1966); and Henry S. Kariel, *The Decline of American Pluralism* (Stanford: Stanford University Press, 1961).

7. One study that uses Bachrach and Baratz's framework in doing this in the area of urban educational policy is Harold B. Savitch, "Powerlessness and Differential Access in New York City," *Polity* 1 (1972): 19-56.

8. See, for example, the differences in the definitions of "primary care" given in Alberta W. Parker, "The Dimensions of Primary Care: Blueprints for Change," in *Primary Care: Where Medicine Fails*, ed. Spyros Andreopoulos (New York: Wiley, 1974), and in Walsh McDermott, "General Medical Care," *Johns Hopkins Medical Journal* 135 (November 1974): 292-321.

9. Staff of the Subcommittee on Health and the Environment of the Committee on Interstate and Foreign Commerce, U.S. House of Representatives, *A Discursive Dictionary of Health Care* (Washington, D.C.: Government Printing Office, 1976), p. 127; emphasis in the original.

10. Peter Bachrach and Morton S. Baratz, *Power and Poverty, Theory and Practice* (New York: Oxford University Press, 1970).

11. Ibid., p. 4.

12. Ibid., p. 7.

13. Ibid., p. 43.

14. Ibid., p. 44.

15. Ibid., pp. 48-49.

16. Ibid., p. 44. Isaac Balbus has made a similar point; see "The Concept of Interests in Pluralist and Marxian Analysis," in *The Politics and Society Reader*, ed. Ira Katznelson et al. (New York: David McKay, 1970), pp. 299-300.

17. See Bachrach and Baratz, *Power and Poverty*, p. 103. It is possible that the shift in the mobilization of bias that they detected was unique in this policy subsystem because, in comparison to other policy areas such as health or housing, antipoverty was one in which few powerful groups had entrenched patterns of vested interests that they wanted to preserve.

18. Ibid., p. 170.

19. Even so, ideology is complicated to measure, and they discuss the shift in the mobilization of bias "in favor of equality of opportunity" (Bachrach and Baratz, *Power and Poverty*, p. 94) in very qualified terms. See ibid., pp. 94-104.

20. Alice Sardell, "The Institutionalization of Reform: An Analysis of Federal Support of Neighborhood Health Centers, 1965-1980" (Ph.D. dissertation, New York University, 1980), chap. 2.

21. See James G. Burrow, *Organized Medicine in the Progressive Era: The Move toward Monopoly* (Baltimore: Johns Hopkins University Press, 1977), pp. 106-113.

22. Charles E. Rosenberg, "Social Class and Medical Care in Nineteenth Century America: The Rise and Fall of the Dispensary," *Journal of the History of Medicine and Allied Sciences* 29 (January 1974):52.

23. John Duffy, *A History of Public Health in New York City, 1866-1966* (New York: Russell Sage Foundation, 1974), pp. 263-267.

24. Ibid., pp. 269-270.

25. Ibid., pp. 270-271.

26. Ibid., pp. 269-270.

27. See George Rosen, "The Idea of Social Medicine in America," *Canadian Medical Association Journal* 61 (September 1949):317-321.

28. This aspect of the health-care system has been dealt with more extensively than the other elements discussed previously. See, for instance, Eliot Friedson, *The Profession of Medicine* (New York: Dodd, Mead, 1972), and idem, *Professional Dominance* (New York: Atherton, 1970).

29. Roger A. Reynolds, "Improving Access to Health Care among the Poor: The Neighborhood Health Center Experience," *The Milbank Memorial Fund Quarterly/Health and Society* 54 (Winter 1976):47.

30. Dr. H. Jack Geiger, interview, New York City, 6 April 1978.

31. Isabel Walsh Pritchard, "Health Care and Reform: The Dilemmas of a Demonstration Program" (Ph.D. dissertation, University of California at Berkeley, 1974), p. 100; emphasis in the original.

32. In addition, the majority of health-center grants went to established health institutions, hospitals, and medical schools in part, so that opposition to the program from these quarters would be prevented. DHEW official, interview, Washington, D.C., 31 March 1978.

33. Geiger interview, 6 April 1978.

34. See Elizabeth J. Anderson et al., *The Neighborhood Health Center Program: Its Growth and Problems* (Washington, D.C.: National Association of Neighborhood Health Centers, Inc., 1976), p. 13.

35. Karen Davis and Cathy Schoen, *Health and the War on Poverty* (Washington, D.C.: Brookings Institution, 1978), p. 164.

36. Richard E. Cairl and Allen W. Imershein, "National Health Insurance Policy in the United States: A Case of Non-Decision-Making," *International Journal of Health Services* 7 (1977):170.

37. Ibid.

38. Ibid., p. 174.

39. Theodore R. Marmor, *The Politics of Medicare* (Chicago: Aldine, 1973), p. 114.

4

Market Reform, Health Systems, and Health Maintenance Organizations

Joseph L. Falkson

This chapter reviews an important contemporary trend in national health policy: the market-reform strategy. The strategy is based on the presumption that the federal role in health affairs for much of the postwar period has been essentially perverse: use of contradictory rather than complementary resource-allocation tools that have promoted conflict among state and local governments, while unsurping their rightful authority; subsidization of hospitals and advanced biomedical technologies to the neglect of alternative health resources; over-commitment to medical specialties to the detriment of community-based general medical practice; third-party, vendor-payment programs uncritically reimbursing hospital and specialized medical services, thereby bloating medicine's pricing structure, eliminating consumer choice from the purchase process, and, generally, exaggerating the need for these services.

While the federal government did not create the sectoral pressures within the nation's health system that maldistributed health-care resources and caused the rapid inflation in health-care costs and prices over the past 20 years, federal-policy responses have exacerbated rather than ameliorated these perverse trends.[1] Federal interventions, involving both subsidies and regulations, have magnified and intensified the internal contradictions of health systems. The critical health-policy questions of the day, therefore, are: How can public authority influence health-systems behavior without aggravating delicately balanced internal relationships among health-system components? How can reforms be initiated without provoking counterproductive reactions?

Origins of Market Reform

A provocative answer to these perplexing questions was taking shape in the late 1960s. Consider Robert A. Levine's analysis:

> The evidence from both domestic and military systems is clearly consistent with the theory that highly administered systems fail with a high probability. . . . Increasingly, . . . economists . . . have . . . turned to the market system that characterizes our American economy for the answer to many problems. . . . The market business system of

the U.S. economy contrasts with a highly administered system because it (1) is decentralized; (2) is self-administered in the sense that most of the prime actors make their own decisions; (3) is motivated by the economic self-interest of these prime actors; (4) requires only the gross application of public policy rather than detailed case-by-case application; (5) is unplanned in the sense of being laid out in advance by external authority.[2]

Charles Schultze, President Carter's chief economic adviser, added his support nearly a decade later:

> Across a wide range of areas, social intervention often fails, not because it relies unnecessarily on regulation or other command-and-control devices, but because in other ways it ignores the roles of properly structured economic incentives for achieving social goals.[3]

Levine and Schultze both recognized the limited capacity of democratic governments in capitalist societies to control the behavior of diverse private markets. They concluded that governmental action worked better where it consciously identified and manipulated incentive structures affecting the behavior of those private markets rather than bypassing them through directly administered bureaucracies. In essence, government ought to expand its reliance on fiscal and monetary policies that make substantial use of private markets, in place of policies requiring complex programs of public management and bureaucratic rule making.

The obvious attraction of market theory is its elimination of reliance on centralized bureaucracies and detailed prescriptions of behavior. The lesson of the 1960s and 1970s has been that the federal government lacks the mechanisms to implement the complex social objectives behind much of the progressive legislation of the past 20 years. There is, however, an essential contradiction that must be addressed: Markets allocate resources according to efficiency criteria, not according to equity criteria. Yet the thrust of much of the progressive health legislation of the past 20 years has been to correct inequities in the availability of health care. Health-care markets failed to produce appropriate types and amounts of health services or distribute them equitably. Why should the nation subsequently turn to this same, flawed marketplace for the remedies previously lacking? How appropriate is the market-reform strategy for reforming health systems?

Market Reform and Health Systems

The critique of federal intervention, on the surface at least, seems to explain many of the failures of recent years in the health sector. Careful analysis of the health system's internal incentive structures clearly discloses that much federal activity has been directed toward isolated cures of symptoms rather than toward comprehensive cures of root problems. For example, the largest federal programs, medicare and medicaid, rapidly accelerated inflationary pressures by supplying health systems with virtually unlimited dollars to pay for expanded population coverage. Health resources were not available in sufficient amounts and in appropriate locations and practice mixes to absorb these expanded entitlements. While solving the accessibility problems of the elderly and poor, on one level, medicare and medicaid drove up the costs of delivering care to all population sectors, on a more profound level.

Similarly, federal efforts to regulate health-resources development gradually evolved from mild attempts to stimulate voluntary self-regulation among private health-care institutions into a full-blown program of mandatory, federally initiated controls on hospital growth. The mandatory program of hospital regulation has had some success in restraining unbridled growth, particularly where services are highly duplicative. In general, however, these regulatory programs have proven to be difficult to administer because they require close monitoring of the health system. Moreover, while significant progress toward bed reduction and hospital mergers can be pointed to, in some locations, this progress owes more to changing demographics and resultant reduced occupancy levels, that is, natural market forces, than to successful regulation.

But if the experiences of federal subsidies and regulations have been disappointing, the appropriateness of a market-reform strategy for rationalizing the behavior of health systems has undergone only limited empirical verification. The impulse of the federal government to tighten its controls over health systems continues with the drive toward mandatory ceilings on price increases.[4] Medicare and medicaid remain essentially passive payers of health-care costs; only recently have incentive-reimbursement experiments been initiated with any consistency.[5] The most consistent experiment has been the 10-year effort to develop prepaid health plans, known as health-maintenance organizations (HMOs). While this effort has fallen far short of original expectations, the experience of HMOs offers cautious optimism for the market-reform advocacy.

HMOs and Market Reform

Ellwood and associates are generally credited with bringing the market-reform strategy of federal intervention to the attention of national health policymakers in 1970.[6] Their contribution was to harmonize market theory with identifiable, alternative health-care-delivery mechanisms known as "prepaid group-practice plans" (PPGPs) and "foundations for medical care" (FMCs).[7] The "health-maintenance strategy" was officially adopted as a cornerstone of national health policy by President Nixon in February of 1971.[8] Quite simply, the plan was to use the power of medicare and medicaid reimbursements to convince physicians to form organized, collective health-service organizations that would receive payment for services on the basis of predetermined prices rather than incurred costs.

If all parties to the medical-care transaction—doctors, hospitals, patients, payers—could agree in advance to the price of a specified range of care, then incentives toward cost efficiency would be created, that is, health-care providers would know that there were only a limited amount of dollars available to cover the costs of providing service. If costs exceeded the fixed-price payment, then providers would have to absorb the loss. Obviously, the fixed-price contract would be a powerful incentive toward restraint in excessive use of costly services such as hospitalization and advanced technology. Coupled with appropriate internal monitoring to ensure that physicians neither used too much nor too little hospital-based services, HMOs could significantly restrain the costs of health care.

Evidence in support of these claims is compelling. For example, the largest PPGP, the Kaiser Health Plans, based predominantly in California, have had a profound impact on hospitalization rates: 349 bed days per 1000 population, annually, compared to an annual national average of 1149 bed days per 1000 population. In essence, the Kaiser plans substitute less expensive visits to doctors in their offices for more expensive hospital stays. In the vast, gray areas of medical care, where physicians have discretion to hospitalize or administer therapy on an outpatient basis, very often the economics of reimbursement will dictate the decision. Where the third-party payer reimburses hospitalization but not office visits, the physician is more likely to hospitalize. He does this both as a gesture to his patient and as a means of assuring payment for himself, that is, hospital insurance usually covers the visits of the admitting physician to the hospital. Moreover, speciality-trained physicians have been drilled to prefer the hospital as the locus for performance of tests and procedures requiring use of technology. Obviously, many such procedures could be performed only in the hospital. But a significant number of routine procedures, for example, X-rays and electrocardiograms, can be safely handled in the outpatient setting. The HMO creates economic incentives that reinforce the choice of the outpatient setting where it is feasible and practical.

The Impulse to Spend and Regulate

The HMO initiative, as originally proposed by the Nixon Administration, focused on the purchasing power of medicare and medicaid to create incentives for the formation of HMOs. Events did not work out quite as they had been planned. For example, the Social Security Administration was ideologically and bureaucratically committed to the cost-reimbursement method of payment. Prepaid, prospective reimbursement, based on a fixed-price service contract,

ominant method of operation of the medicare administration.
ailing cost-reimbursement approach justified an elaborate,
strative apparatus, established to monitor and audit each
d for payment to the Social Security Administration. A
imbursement would eliminate the need for this elaborate
n because HMOs would be allowed a great deal of
ations of their budgets. So long as the HMO remained
determined budget, it would be relatively free to pursue
its progra........ .., .ives without governmental interference.

In a real sense, HMOs challenged the very existence of the medicare bureaucracy. If HMOs worked as they were supposed to, the administrative role of the medicare administration would be greatly contracted. The fact that the prevailing cost-reimbursement system was a major source of inflation was beside the point. Bureaucratic survival was at stake, and the medicare administration successfully resisted efforts to effect a restructuring of the reimbursement mechanism sufficient to accommodate HMOs until 1979. Robbed of the cooperation of medicare, advocates of market reform were forced to seek other ways to promote HMO development.[9] Direct-grant subsidies to HMO developers were undertaken when it became clear the medicare would be an unreliable source of developmental stimulus.

Beginning in 1973 the federal government progressively increased its commitment to HMO development.[10] But federal largesse was not without a significant price: Because HMO development became a special focal point of federal attention, HMOs became the subject of intense regulatory scrutiny. Indeed, the original piece of federal legislation so burdened HMOs with special service and pricing requirements that few developers availed themselves of the opportunity for federal support. The result was exceedingly slow growth in the number of HMOs between 1974-1976. The HMO amendments of 1976, however, deregulated service and pricing requirements in significant ways. Between 1976 and 1979 there were significant increases in the number of operational HMOs.

There are a number of lessons to be drawn from an examination of the federal role in HMO development. First and foremost, there is the lesson of bureaucratic inertia and the great difficulty in getting federal agencies to restrain their enthusiasm for regulation. The federal health bureaucracies fail to distinguish between different levels and types of regulation. The tendency is to develop detailed prescriptions to guide the behavior of health-system components. There has been little recognition of the simple truths that (a) people and institutions will behave the way their self-interest and surrounding incentives lead them, and (b) detailed rules of behavior can easily be subverted where other incentives dictate contrary behavior. No amount of rule making has stymied widespread abuse of the medicare program by unscrupulous physicians. Even honest physicians have found it easy to make less than optimally efficient medical-management decisions.

And yet the federal government clings stubbornly to its discredited approach to reimbursement, with only limited and grudging indulgence of the prepaid, fixed-price approach. Similarly, the federal government insisted on special rules of behavior for federally supported HMOs on the grounds of equity and social justice. However, by requiring HMOs to offer broader benefits and uniform premium coverage to all sectors of the population, without special subsidies, the government was imposing on HMOs burdens that were not required of the non-HMO sectors of health-care systems, thereby threatening the viability of the HMOs. The approach was irrational and self-defeating since it was federal policy to promote HMOs as competitive alternatives to conventional systems of care. Here also we have a graphic illustration of the confusion and contradiction implicit in federal health-care strategies.

A second lesson to be learned is that, just as oppressive regulations can stifle progress, so too can excessive subsidization yield undersirable distortions in health-system growth and development. Thus the twin forces of overregulation and oversubsidization had, by 1980, created a crisis in the HMO industry. A significant number of bankruptcies were being experienced among those HMOs that had relied on substantial federal grants and loans. On the one hand, lavish funding attracted marginal developers with a much higher risk of failure. In earlier years, when funding was much tighter, so too was the screening of potential developers. The result was a lower risk of failure for any given project. On the other hand, these overfunded projects were also burdened with service and pricing requirements that made it difficult for them to compete with conventional insurance plans. The result: failure to achieve financial breakeven and default of federal loans. A realistic approach to regulation and subsidization could have greatly reduced the risk of HMO failures, thereby saving the taxpayers substantial amounts of money. The 1980 congressional-oversight hearings, preparatory to a new round of legislative amendments, promised heated debate over the proprietary of current government HMO policies.

Health Maintenance Organizations and Competition

HMOs perform their mission of cost containment in four ways. First, as already discussed, HMOs create incentives for channeling health-services utilization from costly inpatient settings to less costly outpatient settings. Second, HMOs promote competition with conventional delivery systems, stimulating beneficial responses from these traditional settings. In areas where HMOs have made substantial inroads—San Francisco, Minneapolis, Boston—physicians and hospitals, faced with serious challenges from HMOs, have responded by forming their own prepaid health plans or implementing other cost-containment measures. Third, HMOs have the potential for exercising market power, whereby they are able to obtain preferential prices from various health-care providers. This phenomenon occurs because large HMOs are significant channels of patients to hospitals and, through referrals, to specialty physicians. Finally, a surplus in physician supply is forecast for the 1980s. The natural competitive forces of physicians seeking to hold their patients is already driving many of them to embrace the HMO model.

The Future of Market Reform

Recent trends in the larger national economy underscore a fact often overlooked by health-policy analysts: The health system is part of that larger economy. Double-digit inflation across the board merely reinforces the special vulnerability of the health economy to the perversions robbing it of its dynamism and vitality. From this broader perspective, we can only conclude that the federal government's 10-year romance with HMOs represents a much too timid embrace of the market-reform approach. Ironically, HMOs have been forced to carry the entire burden of reforming health-care markets, shackled with unfair regulatory scrutiny, while conventional cost-reimbursing private health insurance operates under no similar limitations.

The positive although limited experiences of HMOs ought to provide hesitant lawmakers with sufficient evidence to begin expansion of market-reform incentives into the larger health system. One significant step would be to reexamine the preferential, tax-exempt treatment afforded the voluntary health-insurance plans (that is, Blue Cross/Blue Shield). These plans dominate the conventional insurance market. Their superior market power coupled with tax-exempt status enables Blue Cross/Blue Shield plans to block competition effectively. The smaller segment of the insurance market, controlled by commercial, profit-making plans, as well as HMOs, have trouble developing premiums that can compete with Blue Cross/Blue Shield plans because part of their costs are being unfairly subsidized by the federal tax systems. Removal of this anticompetitive advantage would allow HMOs and commercial insurers to compete effectively against Blue Cross/Blue Shield and seriously challenge their superior market power. True price competition would result, to the benefit of the health-care consumer.

In a similar vein, HMOs must be unburdened of onerous federal regulatory controls. Their benefit packages must be allowed to compete with conventional insurance benefits. Community rating, which requires HMOs to charge uniform rates to all segments of the community, provides an unfair competitive advantage to conventional health insurers who can experience rate, that is, adjust premiums to utilization experiences. While equity considerations are important public-policy matters, it is unfair to force HMOs to community rate, while allowing the dominant, conventional insurers to experience rate. The solution would be either to allow HMOs to experience rate or—better still—force all insurers to community rate.

These and other reforms would move the health system a long way toward true competition. The present system is uncompetitive because powerful, vested interests are protected by tradition, biased federal subsidies, and protective regulations, unfairly administered by captive public bureaucracies.

Promotion of market reform has been thwarted by reactionary forces which in other settings have loudly derived loss of freedom to federal encroachment. Barriers to competition are retained in the name of equity. But the search for equity is obstructed by the economic inefficiency of entrenched privilege. Only when these privileges are removed and health-care providers are forced to compete with each other will true economic sovereignty be restored to the health-care consumer. Such sovereignty is the only true equity.

Notes

1. See Joseph L. Falkson, *HMOs and the Politics Health System Reform* (Chicago: American Hospital Association, 1980), pp. 1-3, 23-25, for further discussion of contradictory health programs and the federal role in promoting them.

2. Robert A. Levine, *Public Planning: Failure and Redirection* (New York: Basic Books, 1972), p. 19.

3. Charles L. Schultze, *The Public Use of Private Interest* (Washington, D.C.: The Brookings Institution, 1977), p. 63.

4. The Carter administration introduced a mandatory hospital cost-containment measure on two occasions, only to be rejected by Congress.

5. Although the original medicare legislation that went into effect in 1966 provided authority to experiment with alternative methods of reimbursement, the authority was seldom used. Only after the medicare program was removed from the Social Security Administration and placed within a new agency, the Health Care Financing Administration (HCFA), in 1977, did significant experimentation begin.

6. Paul M. Ellwood, Jr., M.D. is president of the Minneapolis-based health-policy thinktank, InterStudy.

7. Prepaid group-practice plans (PPGPs) are organized groups of physicians, usually working under the same roof, who receive salaries or partnership drawn from a pool of revenues derived from fixed-price premiums charged to subscribers on an annual basis. Foundations for Medical Care (FMCs) served as models for "individual practice associations" (IPAs), which organized reimbursement of solo-practice physicians out of a fixed-price revenue pool. Individual physicians may be reimbursed on a fee-for-service or percentage-of-capitation method. PPGPs and FMCs differ in the degree of structure and control they impose upon physicians. In general, FMCs and IPAs are more flexible in their tolerance of practice pattern organization.

8. Richard M. Nixon, "National Health Strategy," the White House, 18 February 1971.

9. Subsequent to the early rebuff of HMO, the medicare administration sharply limited the possibility of Title 18 or Title 19 (medicare or medicaid) HMOs develop by creating the "50-50" rule. It required that HMOs could not have aggregate enrollments of more than 50 percent medicare or medicaid enrollees also enrolled in an HMO. This regulation severely limited the availability of HMOs to the poor and the elderly.

10. The HMO Act of 1973, PL 93-222, authorized that new starts be developed through the award of federal grants-in-aid.

Part III
Planning and Regulation

5

Prospective Reimbursement of Hospital Costs: Current Developments and Future Prospects

James M. Cameron

Inflation is viewed by the vast majority of Americans as the single most important domestic problem. The cost of medical care, which during the past decade and a half has risen faster than most other sectors of the economy, currently accounts for 9 percent of the gross national product (GNP). As a greater proportion of the nation's resources are spent on medical care, fewer resources are available for other needs. Since the enactment of medicare and medicaid in the mid-1960s, hospital costs have risen at a rate faster than other components of medical-care services. In 1979 hospital costs accounted for approximately 45 percent of total personal-health-care expenditures; government—federal, state, and local—paid for over half of the cost of hospital care.[1] For the most part, hospital care is provided under nonmarket conditions. In a market system those who demand, consume, and pay for a product or service are the same. In the hospital-care marketplace, all three are different entities—physicians demand, patients consume, and third parties pay. A market implies competitive conditions among providers that has an effect on price. There does exist competition within the hospital industry—competition among hospitals for physicans to serve on their medical staffs and admit patients to fill their beds—but the only effect it has on price is to drive it upward.[2]

The unrestrained rise in hospital costs coupled with expanded federal financing has led to the creation of three basic types of governmental control programs aimed at curbing the rise in hospital costs: (1) control of capital investment, (2) control of utilization, and (3) control of reimbursement.

The first two governmental control efforts to contain hospital costs have not been encouraging. With the enactment of the National Health Planning and Resources Development Act of 1974, approval of major capital investments must be made by the state certificate-of-need agency after initial recommendation by the local health-systems agency. Early evidence suggests that the success of certificate-of-need controls has been limited at best. Studies have found that certificate of need has not had a significant effect on the level of plant assets or on total hospital investment.[3] The federal initiative in 1972 to create Professional Standards Review Organizations (PSROs) reflected an attempt to reduce unnecessary medical procedures and length of hospital stays. The PSRO utilization-review activities include approving admissions, determining appropriate lengths of stay, and certifying extensions of the initial lengths of stay. For the most part, the program has not been found to be cost effective.[4] The PSRO program, which relies on the authority of local physicians, may provide inadequate incentives to constrain the utilization of hospital services.

The third type of governmental effort, control of reimbursement through prospective payment systems, may offer more promise for controlling hospital costs. A growing number of policymakers have come to believe that the prevailing methods of retrospective reimbursement provide incentives for overutilization of hospital services. Prospective reimbursement,[5] in which payment rates are set in advance, is designed to offer direct incentives for hospitals to control expenditures. In spite of the formidable resistance to further regulation of the hospital industry, prospective reimbursement, as a means of moderating hospital-cost inflation, is quickly gaining currency among state and federal policymakers.

Retrospective Reimbursement

The absence of normal market mechanisms that might serve to induce efficiencies in the delivery of hospital care is exacerbated by the system of reimbursement. Hospital reimbursement is currently a complex, fractionalized system, characterized by inequities among purchasers of care (patients and their third-party payers) and perverse incentives for the providers of care (hospitals and their physicians). Fractionalization results primarily from varying payment arrangements among hospitals and payers—medicare, medicaid, Blue Cross plans, and commercial insurance/self-pay. The various payers not only have different bases for payment but within a payor class the basis for payment may differ from region to region.

In order to appreciate the challenge faced by policymakers concerned with reforming hospital-reimbursement policy, it is necessary to disentangle the current system of retrospective reimbursement and examine some of its effects on hospital-cost inflation. There are two central issues to be addressed in identifying the basis on which hospitals are reimbursed: (1) What are the financial elements for which the hospital is paid, and how is the hospital paid?

With respect to *what* the hospital is paid for, medicare and medicaid (under Titles 18 and 19 of the Social Security Act) pay hospitals for the operating costs incurred in treating their own patients. That is, while hospitals will recover from federal payers that portion of hospital operating costs, (salaries, supplies, and depreciation) consumed by medicare and medicaid patients, hospitals will not recover other financial requirements common to any business enterprise. These include expenses associated with the provision of care to patients for whom no one pays (charity care and bad debts) and replacement costs of capital facilities in excess of historical depreciation. For many Blue Cross plans, reimbursement is patterned similar to the federal payers, while other Blue Cross plans may pay for a portion of some or all of these additional financial requirements. The financial elements covered by Blue Cross plans vary depending on the provider contract negotiated with hospitals in each service area.[6] Commercial insurers and self-pay patients reimburse hospitals at rates determined by the hospitals themselves; these include not only the operating costs associated with treating these patients (and their proportionate share of the additional financial requirements) but also the portion of financial requirements not borne by medicare, medicaid, and Blue Cross. Hospitals often set rates for these patients to also allow for a return on equity.

Thus for the same hospital services, there exists an unequal distribution across multiple payers with respect to what financial elements are reimbursed. None of these reimbursement arrangements provide incentives for delivering hospital services efficiently. Moreover, the fragmented reimbursement system has contributed to severe financial hardship for many innercity hospitals, which often have a high percentage of patients who are not covered by insurance but who nevertheless are unable or unwilling to pay their hospital bills. Depleting their capital reserves in order to cover their normal operating costs, these hospitals often have insufficient capital to replace deteriorating or obsolete plant and equipment.[7]

With respect to *how* the hospital is paid, two methods of reimbursement predominate. The per-diem method of reimbursement, typified by medicare and most medicaid programs and Blue Cross plans, entails setting an interim payment rate in advance of the fiscal year. This is established by dividing the payer's total hospital costs (of the previous fiscal year) by that payer's patient days and adjusting for inflation. This interim per-diem rate is adjusted at year end to the actual costs incurred. A second method of reimbursement consists of itemized charges for the specific services delivered to each patient ("menu of charges"). While commercial insurers, self-pay patients, and a few Blue Cross plans pay these actual charges, many medicaid programs and some Blue Cross plans pay a percentage of charges (adjusted to actual cost at year end).

The immediate incentives for the hospital with respect to per-diem reimbursement is to increase patient days (that is, length of stay). Reimbursement on the basis of a menu of charges provides hospitals with immediate incentives to increase the volume of services delivered and to increase the charges for those services more typically consumed by charge-based payors' patients. Neither type of payment unit—per diem or menu of charges—offers incentives for containing hospital costs.

The openended nature of retroactive, cost-based reimbursement encourages hospitals and their physicians to expand the volume and intensity of service without concern for cost. Hospitals are reimbursed for a production process that is inherently inflationary. "To ensure their financial viability and growth they have adopted and become quite effective at producing the product defined by the reimbursement mechanism—cost and patient days."[8] By defining a hospital's "product" in terms of inputs—costs or days of stay—hospital behavior is oriented toward maximizing expenses in order to maximize revenues. Hospital administrators find that they must "game" the reimbursement system in order to maximize revenues. Gaming the reimbursement system involves setting differential itemized charges depending on (1) the mix of payers, (2) the process of determining costs, and (3) the unit of payment associated with each payer. At bottom, the financial health of a hospital depends more on the administrator's ability to maximize reimbursement than on efforts to improve the efficiency with which services are delivered.

Prospective Reimbursement Programs

Prospective reimbursement, in which payment rates are set in advance of the period over which they are to apply, is widely advocated as a mechanism for inducing hospitals to be more efficient. In contrast to traditional retrospective reimbursement, a prospective payment system involves an external body in determining rates and offers incentives for hospitals to control expenditures so as not to exceed their prospective rates. There are several rate-regulation approaches including hospital-by-hospital review and negotiation of budgets, budget review by exception in which cost screens are employed to identify unacceptable increases in costs, and formula methods that use statistical formulas to establish allowable unit costs and allowable rate increases.

Prospective reimbursement programs have been initiated by a number of Blue Cross plans and hospital associations. Hospital participation in these programs has been on a voluntary basis, however, and they usually have not applied to medicare and medicaid. Several states have legislated programs requiring review or regulation of hospital rates and budgets. Although the purpose of all these programs has been to provide an acceptable method of constraining the rise in hospital rates, they vary significantly in the type of administrative body in which they are based, degree of compliance required, program methodology, payers covered, frequency of review and appeals procedures.

Two states whose prospective reimbursement programs have generated considerable interest over the past few years, Rhode Island and New York, illustrate quite different approaches to rate setting. Rhode Island's prospective rate-setting system entails a negotiation process between third-party payers (Blue Cross and medicaid) and the Hospital Association of Rhode Island, under the aegis of the state budget office, to set a limit on total allowable operating expense increases in the state during the coming year. Each hospital subsequently negotiates its budget with the third parties, focusing on incremental changes (including inflation, volume changes, and approved new and expanded services) from current to prospective years. The strong role of Blue Cross in the program and the small number of hospitals involved have contributed to the success of the program. Although in fiscal year 1975, the first year of the program, the actual increase in hospital expenditures was not significantly below the national average, fiscal years 1976 through 1979 witnessed actual increases well below the national average. The state of New York has had a prospective reimbursement system since 1970 based on statistical formulas for Blue Cross and medicaid plans with no retroactive adjustment (although it does allow for a hospital to appeal its rate after the prospective year). After grouping hospitals by similar characteristics, the statistical formulas compare costs and patient days of each hospital within its peer group. Studies of the cost-containment effort in New York suggest that the program has been successful in slowing the increase in hospital expenditures.[9] Evaluations of prospective rate-setting programs in other states have also reported some degree of cost savings relative to the nation as a whole.[10] Although these studies are inconclusive, the available evidence suggests that prospective reimbursement may have a positive impact on controlling hospital costs. In fact, as shown in table 5-1, for the past few years the rate of increase in hospital expenses for those states with mandatory prospective reimbursement systems has been significantly lower than for those states without mandatory controls on hospital rates.

Although these state programs may have contributed to holding down hospital-cost inflation, prospective reimbursement systems in the 1970s did little to alter the basic structure of third-party payment. Prospective reimbursement programs have in a sense been layered on top of the existing, fragmented hospital-reimbursement system. Prospective rates have typically been

Table 5-1
Percent Increases in Community-Hospital Expenses

	Number of Hospitals	1976-1977	1977-1978	1978-1979
Massachusetts	117	13.7	7.1	9.6
Rhode Island	14	10.9	8.6	11.7
Connecticut	36	11.3	10.6	9.9
New York	288	6.2	7.1	10.1
New Jersey	104	11.9	9.2	11.4
Maryland	53	11.8	12.2	14.8
Washington	108	15.1	11.6	12.9
Total for states with mandatory prospective reimbursement programs	720	9.5	8.3	10.7
All other states	5131	15.7	14.0	14.2
United States	5851	14.2	12.6	13.4

Source: American Hospital Association, *Hospital Statistics,* 1977, 1978, 1979, and 1980 editions, table 5c.

established on the basis of cost, without reference to additional financial requirements. In some states, especially New York, this has contributed to large deficits for many innercity hospitals.[11] These hospitals have had trouble accommodating themselves to cost-based prospective payment systems because of the nature of their patient populations and the inability to generate adequate capital to meet their financial requirements. With a steadily decreasing percentage of charge-paying patients, the patient population of these hospitals has become predominately medicare, medicaid, and patients unable to pay their hospital bills. Reimbursement for capital assets by federal payers has been based on historical cost depreciation. With inflation, historical cost depreciation provides insufficient funds to cover current and future capital requirements.[12] Lacking adequate formation of capital, and faced with growing deficits, many innercity hospitals have been forced to close. As the principal source of health care for the poor and medically indigent, others have remained open, subsidized by local government. The financial hardships experienced by many public general hospitals under prospective reimbursement programs may have had a negative impact on both the quality of and access to care for the poor.

Another troublesome aspect of prospective reimbursement systems has been the basis for determining the unit of payment. Cost comparisons among hospitals, and year-end adjustments for volume, have been made on a per-diem or menu-of-charges basis, thus retaining a structure of incentives that may discourage decreases in lengths of stay or intensity of services. The inability of such crude measures of output (per diem or units of service) to reflect the uniqueness of individual hospitals has in many instances led to successful appeals to the prospective rates initially proposed by the rate-setting agencies. Peer grouping, an effort to classify hospitals on the basis of similar characteristics, has lacked sufficient sensitivity to account for differences in cost. In addition, comparing hospitals on the basis of cost per patient day or cost per unit of service does not adequately account for or encourage efficiencies in the delivery of care. These problems have resulted from the lack of a definition of hospital output; that is, the ability to measure sufficiently patient case mix. In their examination of the central issues related to regulation, the American Hospital Association argued that the regulation of hospital rates should explicitly recognize patient case mix "because only in this way can the relative efficiency of hospitals be evaluated."[13]

The problem of fractionalization has not been alleviated and in some cases has been aggrevated by focusing the prospective rate-setting effort on a portion of the payers only. The inequities among payers with respect to the amount paid for the same services has increased in most states with mandatory prospective rate setting.[14]

The early development of prospective rate setting reflected locally initiated, piecemeal efforts. Set within the existing framework of cost-based reimbursement, prospective rate-setting methodologies did little to redress inequities among payers nor were they able to adequately account for differences among hospitals. In addition to methodological difficulties, mandatory prospective reimbursement systems have usually been initiated in the face of stiff political opposition from the hospital industry, often limiting program effectiveness. In spite of hospital opposition to government intervention in the rate-setting process, prospective reimbursement has become increasingly attractive to policy-makers. Interest in prospective reimbursement has been augmented by the recent role of the federal government. The implementation of Section 222 of PL 92-603, amendments to the Social Security Act, provided federal funding for prospective reimbursement experiments and allowed for the inclusion of medicare patients in prospective reimbursement systems. The federal government thereby entered the prospective reimbursement arena providing a major spur to the development of more sophisticated methodologies and further legitimizing prospective reimbursement as a potential solution to the problem of hospital cost containment. In 1976 and 1977 seven HEW contracts were awarded for experimental development of prospective reimbursement systems— New Jersey, Maryland, Connecticut, Massachusetts, Blue Cross of Western Pennsylvania, and the Finger Lakes Health Systems Agency (Rochester, New York).

Commensurate with the implementation of these federally funded experiments, a number of recent trends in prospective reimbursement can be discerned. As indicated previously, basing rate setting solely on costs may have exacerbated the financial difficulties of many innercity hospitals and led to greater problems of access to care for the poor and medically indigent. Recently some states have used prospective reimbursement as a vehicle to address these problems by directing the focus of attention in rate setting to net revenues rather than expenses. There appears to be an emerging trend to set rates on the basis of an equitable set of financial requirements for *all* payers. Another trend has been the establishment of independent rate-setting commissions; this tends to remove the locus of regulation from the traditional state health bureaucracy and has the effect of expediting appeals procedure.

Probably the most significant development in prospective reimbursement is the emergence of a feasible and statistically valid method of measuring hospital case mix. Utilizing a hospital patient-classification scheme comprised of homogenous patient groups, a few states have begun to set prospective hospital rates that explicitly account for the types of patients treated.

Current Developments

Two states with mandatory prospective reimbursement systems that best exemplify these recent trends are Maryland and New Jersey. Although prospective rate setting began for both states in the mid-1970s, truly innovative approaches that have come to grips with the problem of fragmentation of the reimbursement system have occurred only recently. For the two states the road to development of a new approach to prospective reimbursement has been different not only in the development of rate-setting methodologies but with respect to the political environment within which the policy innovations were developed and implemented.

Maryland

From the outset the Maryland Hospital Association (MHA) has had a central role in the initiation and development of prospective rate setting. In the early 1970s the legislature passed a prospective reimbursement law, proposed by the MHA, that established the Health Services Cost Review Commission (HSCRC). In addition to providing a framework for a governmental role in hospital cost control, the law provided that all nonfederal payers assume equitably the reasonable financial requirements of hospitals.

The hospital associations of nearly all other states have been adamantly opposed to government regulation of hospital rates; yet in Maryland the hospital association led the way in establishing a state agency with the power to approve or deny a hospital's rates. The MHA already had in place a voluntary prospective review of hospital budgets, but it had had little success in holding down costs. In an atmosphere of strong public support for legislative action to help curb the rise in hospital costs, the MHA decided to influence its formulation rather than attempt to oppose it.[15] The prospect of a government-centered cost-control effort was, for MHA, an acceptable trade-off for a law that would promote the financial solvency of hospitals, many of which were moving toward bankruptcy. Maryland's innercity hospitals had been experiencing severe deficits resulting from two interrelated factors. First, as with many other cities on the East Coast, the declining economic base of Maryland's cities, particularly Baltimore, had led to a change in hospital caseload to one more heavily comprised of patients on cost-based federal reimbursement or charity and bad debts. Second, Blue Cross represented a larger share of the hospital insurance market in Maryland than it did for most other states. Like medicare and medicaid, the Maryland Blue Cross plan paid only the costs associated with treating its own patients resulting in an unusually large cost-to-charge differential. Hospitals were therefore forced to spend an increasing portion of their capital-depreciation funds in order to meet the costs of treating the medically indigent. This left little or no money for capital replacement, which in turn led to further hospital deterioration.

The HSCRC began to set prospective rates in July of 1974 for Blue Cross and commercial/self-pay patients. For Blue Cross this meant that it would share in paying for bad debts and capital-replacement costs. In July of 1977, after obtaining a federal prospective reimbursement contract allowing for a medicare and medicaid waiver,[16] the HSCRC began to set prospective rates for federal payers as well. Thus the commission established a uniform basis across all payers, for determining what financial elements hospitals would be paid for. The rate for each payer consisted of its share not only of operating costs but also its share of bad debts and capital-replacement costs. The prospective reimbursement system was designed to limit the growth of operating costs, thereby freeing up additional resources to meet other critical financial requirements of hospitals. This improved the prospects for the financial health of many innercity hospitals that might otherwise have been forced to close.

The HSCRC set prospective rates through a process of budget review focusing on rates of increase for departmental units of service.[17] Approved rates per unit of service were derived from comparisons with similar hospitals and other criteria, subject to negotiation and appeal. The rate-setting procedures, although moderating per-unit cost increases, provided no incentives for holding down increases in service intensity. With respect to *how* hospitals were reimbursed, therefore, the system reflected some of the flaws of retrospective cost reimbursement. In spite of a provision in the regulations aimed at minimizing the incentives for hospitals to increase service intensity—a volume-variance adjustment whereby hospitals would recover the costs associated with volume increase but would not profit from them—the commission found that intensity of services nevertheless continued to increase. The heart of the problem seemed to lie in the continued focus on units of service—hospital inputs—rather than the medical case treated—hospital outputs.

In an attempt to meet head on the issue of incentives for the reduction of service intensity, the commission in 1976 piloted a "Guaranteed Inpatient Revenue" (GIR) system, on a voluntary basis, with a few large teaching hospitals. GIR involves determining a guaranteed amount of revenue per inpatient admission that the hospital can collect during the course of the prospective year.[18] It provides a financial incentive to reduce the intensity of services (that is, units of service per patient), while retaining incentives to reduce the cost of delivering each unit of service. Hospitals for which actual revenues received are less than their guaranteed revenues per admission will receive the difference in the following year's rates. The guaranteed-inpatient-revenue amount is tied to the hospital's reasonable costs, which in turn had been determined on the basis of the system of budget review referred to earlier. The GIR is annually adjusted to account for inflation, a 1-percent service-intensity factor,[19] and changes in patient case mix. Under this sytem, the inflation-adjusted reasonable costs of a GIR hospital in a given base year will increase 1 percent per year if the hospital continues to treat the same volume and mix of patients. The HSCRC has experimented with various methods of monitoring case-mix changes related to diagnostic type and payer class. The GIR system is currently applied to fifteen Maryland hospitals (including all hospitals with over 400 beds).

Preliminary results for 1979 show that although expenses for all hospitals in Maryland increased at a rate slightly higher than the national average,[20] GIR hospitals experienced increases almost 3 percent less than the non-GIR hospitals.[21] The system, designed to offer concrete incentives for more efficient utilization of hospital resources, appears to be successfully controlling hospital-cost inflation, while simultaneously providing adequate resources for hospitals to meet their financial requirements. The Maryland HSCRC has addressed directly the question of what financial elements purchasers of care will reimburse: All payors pay equitably for operating costs, uncompensated-care costs, capital-replacement costs, and working-capital costs. Furthermore, they have addressed directly the question of how rates should be structured and payments made in order to induce appropriate incentives to hospitals and their physicians.

New Jersey

Whereas in Maryland the hospital association was instrumental in the adoption of a mandatory prospective reimbursement system, hospitals in New Jersey have adamently opposed a governmental role in hospital cost containment. In 1971 the legislature gave the state Department of Health the fiat to review hospital costs and to set prospective rates for certain payers. However, the state neglected to exercise this authority and relied instead upon the New Jersey Hospital Association (NJHA) to assume the responsibility for cost containment. Increasing disenchantment with NJHA's voluntary budget-review system finally led the state Department of Health to implement the Standard Hospital Accounting and Rate Evaluation (SHARE) System—a prospective budget-review process imposing mandatory limits on per-diem payment rates for Blue Cross and medicaid patients.[22] The state's entry into the cost-containment arena signaled the beginning of vigorous opposition by hospitals to governmental involvement in hospital reimbursement.

The state's prospective reimbursement effort, although directed toward curbing the rise in hospital costs, neglected the interrelated problem of differential reimbursement principles across payers. Insofar as the system applied to only Blue Cross and medicaid and did not alter the determination of what financial elements each payer included in its rates (neither payer reimbursed hospitals for uncompensated-care and capital-replacement costs), the financial troubles of innercity hospitals were exacerbated. As in Maryland, urban areas in New Jersey were experiencing a rapidly declining economic base, and Blue Cross, representing a very high proportion of privately insured patients, paid only the cost of treating its own patients. The plight of New Jersey's innercity hospitals was even more grave than conditions in Maryland; however, since medicaid in New Jersey covered only the categorically needy, eschewing coverage of the medically indigent. Although the SHARE system may have slowed the rise in hospital expenses (see table 5-1), it tended to aggravate the financial problems of innercity hospitals. These hospitals were typically older institutions serving primarily lower income patients. Revenues derived from the relatively small proportion of charge-paying patients and declining philanthropic donations were insufficient to offset losses in revenues associated with bad debts coupled with the restrictions of the SHARE rate-setting system. Many hospitals were thereby forced to utilize depreciation funds for their day-to-day operations rather than applying these funds toward replacement of obsolete facilities and equipment.

With respect to how rates were set, the SHARE system was based on cost per patient day. The focus on per-diem costs had little or no effect on reducing lenghts of stay, nor did it offer adequate incentives for slowing the rise in ancillary-service utilization. In addition, the use of patient days as the mechanism for measuring hospital efficiency augmented opposition to the SHARE system by hospitals that contended that the system did not recognize differences in patient case mix.

Within a year after the initiation of the SHARE system, the Department of Health applied for and received HEW funding for a prospective reimbursement experiment based on patient case mix.[23] As with the Maryland GIR system, the New Jersey experiment was designed to reverse the existing structure of incentives such that hospitals could maximize net income through reductions in per-patient costs. The New Jersey prospective reimbursement experiment utilized a recently developed patient-classification system that defines hospital products in terms of a manageable number of homogenous patient classes, called Diagnosis-Related Groups (DRGs).[24] The DRG patient-classification system provides the basis for setting per-case prospective rates.

Developmental work on the DRG prospective reimbursement experiment began in late 1976 and came to fruition in January of 1980 with the setting of mandatory prospective rates for each of the 383 DRGs for 26 hospitals. The controversial rate-setting system traveled a tortuous road to implementation. Many hospital administrators familiar with the DRG experiment believed that the system encompassed a fairer basis of comparison for judging the costs of treating their mix of patients than the SHARE system. Nevertheless, the hospitals' distrust of state regulation, largely resulting from their experience with the SHARE prospective rate-setting system, was augmented by the incipient implementation of the DRG prospective reimbursement experiment. Because the system applied to all payers, it represented far greater regulatory control over hospital behavior. Furthermore, the uncertainty associated with the novel, technically complex regulatory system contributed to hospital resistance to the system. The NJHA conducted a well-organized effort to thwart the implementation of a rate-setting system based on patient case mix. However, the impending bankruptcy of many of the NJHA's innercity members produced a split within the organization. The financially troubled hospitals stood to benefit substantially from legislation prescribing prospective rate setting for all payers based on the full financial requirements of hospitals. Ultimately, NJHA aquiesced to the new legislation. In order to implement the legislative mandate and simultaneously comply with federal requirements regarding rate setting applied to medicare patients, the state Department of Health adopted a mandatory prospective reimbursement system based on the DRG experiment methodology.

Reimbursement based on patient case mix represents a radical departure from earlier prospective reimbursement systems. Rather than being paid on the basis of charges or per diem, hospitals bill patients and third-party payers by the type of medical case (that is, the specific DRG). The use of DRGs provides the basis for identifying a common unit of output and a readily comparable price for patient care. Since hospitals are reimbursed on the basis of their DRG-specific performance relative to other hospitals, the system appears to offer a market-like competitive context for the provision of patient care.

Implications for the Future

Implementing reimbursement reform in Maryland and New Jersey has involved considerable political turmoil—opposition from the hospital industry (particularly in New Jersey), long legal battles, bureaucratic infighting, and incessant conflict among planning and regulating bodies. These new systems, however, may represent the "cutting edge" of policy innovation in the area of prospective reimbursement. Maryland's GIR system and New Jersey's system based on patient case mix deal directly with the two most important issues related to fragmentation of the reimbursement system—what financial elements payers are responsible for and how payment rates are to be set. Both systems utilize the DRG patient-classification scheme to identify hospital case mix, although it is employed somewhat differently. Whereas the Maryland GIR system sets a hospital's rates based on changes in its own case mix, the New Jersey system sets a hospital's rates based on DRG-specific comparisons with other hospitals (and requires that participating hospitals actually bill on a per-case basis).

The DRGs provide the foundation for a "common language" among the patient, the physican, and third-party payers. In addition, they provide the potential for directly involving the physician with the financial consequences of his use of hospital resources. The concept of regulating hospital costs on the basis of case mix may serve to encourage the development of a competitive environment. In the New Jersey system hospitals are compared with each other on the basis of a common unit of output. There is therefore a built-in incentive for a hospital to attempt to produce the same "product" at a lower cost. The hospital stands to gain if its costs fall below that of other hospitals.

The innovative approaches to prospective reimbursement in Maryland and New Jersey have begun to attract considerable interest among other states that are examining alternative methods for confronting the problem of hospital inflation.[25] The federal government, which has funded several prospective reimbursement demonstration projects, also appears to be preparing for the eventual implementation of some form of prospective rate-setting methodology to be applied to all federally insured patients. A preliminary step is the requirement that hospitals submit an annual hospital report that provides for a uniform method of accounting and reporting.[26] Federal interest in the DRG methodology, as a way of specifying and comparing differences in hospitals' case mix, is reflected in recent proposals for setting total cost limits for medicare patients using DRGs.[27] Whether or not the federal government ultimately adopts a prospective reimbursement system similar to the Maryland or New Jersey systems, it is clear that the focus of attention with respect to innovation in prospective reimbursement is turning to the experience of these two states.

Notes

1. Health Care Financing Administration, *Health Care Financing Trends* 1 (Spring 1980).

2. Much of the health-economics literature focuses on market failure in the health sector and the effects on cost. For a clear incisive analysis, see Joseph P. Newhouse, *The Economics of Medical Care: A Policy Perspective* (Reading, Mass.: Addison-Wesley, 1978).

3. Fred Hellinger, "The Effect of Certificate-of-Need Legislation on Hospital Investment," *Inquiry* 13 (Summer 1976): 187-193; David S. Salkever and Thomas Bice, *Hospital Certificate-of-Need Controls: Impact on Investment, Costs, and Use* (Washington, D.C.: American Enterprize Institute, 1979).

4. Robert Brook, et al, *Controlling the Use and Cost of Medical Services: The New Mexico Experimental Medical Care Review Organization—A Four Year Case Study* (Santa Monica: The Rand Corporation, 1978); A. Dobson, et al, "PPSROs: Their Current Status and Their Impact to Date," *Inquiry* 15 (Summer 1978); Richard Averill and Laurence McMahon, "A Cost Benefit Analysis of Continued Stay Certification," *Medical Care* 15 (February 1977): 158-173; see also P.M. Gertman et al, "Summary and Discussion of Findings," *Medical Care* 17 (August 1979):96-103, who suggest that PSROs may have had some small beneficial effect, but stress that all retrospective evaluations of PSROs face serious methodological problems.

5. The term "prospective reimbursement" is somewhat incorrect since it actually refers to prospective "payment"; however, insofar as the approach is generally called prospective reimbursement, it will be referred to as such in this chapter.

6. Blue Cross provider contracts also differ with respect to the method of calculating operating costs for Blue Cross's patients (referred to as "cost finding"). In some cases the cost-finding process is the same as medicare and medicaid; in others it is quite different.

7. A growing body of literature focusing on the problems of public general hospitals has emerged recently. For a good overview of the different approaches analysts have taken in examining the problems as prospects for financially troubled hospitals; see Eli Ginzberg, Michael L. Millman, and Charles Brecher, "The Problematic Future of Public General Hospitals," *Health and Medical Care Services Review* 2 (Summer 1979): 1-11; see also David W. Goff, "The Plight of the Urban Public Hospital," *Journal of Health Politics, Policy and Law* 4 (Winter 1980):657-674.

8. Charles R. Buck, Jr., "Hospitals Produce What They Are Paid For: Costs and Patient Days," *Health Care Management Review* 2 (Fall 1977): 59.

9. Ralph E. Berry, "Prospective Rate Reimbursement and Cost Containment: Formula Reimbursement in New York," *Inquiry* 13 (September 1976): 288-301; Fred J. Hellinger, "An Empirical Analysis of Several Prospective Reimbursement Systems," in Michael Zubkoff, et al (eds.), *Hospital Cost Containment; Selected Notes for Future Policy* (New York: Milbank Memorial Fund, 1978), pp. 370-400.

10. Clifton R. Gaus and Fred J. Hellinger, "Results of Prospective Reimbursement", *Topics in Health Care Financing* 3 (Winter 1976):83-96; William L. Dowling, Hospital Rate-Setting Programs: How, and How Well, Do They Work?" *Topics in Health Care Financing* 6 (Fall 1979):15-22.

11. Nora Piore, Purlaine Lieberman, and James Linnane, "Public Expenditures and Private Control? Health Care Dilemmas in New York City," *Milbank Memorial Fund Quarterly* 55 (Winter 1977):97-116.

12. William O. Cleverley, "Reimbursement for Capital Costs," *Topics in Health Care Financing* 6 (Fall 1979):127-139; Stuart O. Schweitzer, John A. Holder, and Jan H. Ouren, "Reimbursement for Health Facility Capital Formation," paper presented at the Health Capital Conference, Johns Hopkins University, Baltimore, Maryland, 19 February 1980.

13. American Hospital Association, *Hospital Regulation: Report of the Special Committee on the Regulatory Process* (Chicago: American Hospital Association, 1977).

14. For example, the relatively low rate of increase for cost-based payers in Rhode Island and New York during fiscal years 1977, 1978, and 1979 (table 5-1) may be compared with the relatively uncontrolled rates for charge payers. For Rhode Island, the increases in charges to commercially insured and self-pay patients were 13.3 percent in 1977, 11.4 percent in 1978, and 13.2 percent in 1979; for New York the increases were 12.2 percent, 10.1 percent, and 10.5 percent, respectively. These increases for commercially insured and self-pay patients were substantially higher than the rates of increase of cost-based payers.

15. Arnold H. Raphaelson and Charles P. Hall, Jr., "Politics and Economics of Hospital Cost Containment," *Journal of Health Politics, Policy and Law* 3 (Spring 1978):87-111.

16. The Health Care Financing Administration of DHHS has maintained that waivers from "reasonable cost" retrospective reimbursement for medicare patients would only be approved for federally funded prospective reimbursement experiments; furthermore, it must be demonstrated that medicare payments would be less than would otherwise have been paid.

17. Maryland Hospital Education Institute, *A Guide to Rate Review in Maryland Hospitals*, Vol. 1 (Lutherville, Md.: MHEI, 1978); see also U.S. Department of Health Education and Welfare, *National Hospital Rate-Setting Study, Vol. III: Case Study of Prospective Reimbursement in Maryland*, Health Care Financing Grants and Contracts Report, Health Care Financing Administration, April 1980.

18. Maryland Hospital Education Institute, *A Guide to Rate Review in Maryland Hospitals, Vol. 2: The Guaranteed Inpatient Revenue System* (Lutherville, Md.: MHEI, 1979).

19. The "service-intensity factor" refers to an allowance in addition to inflation increases to be used to upgrade services and facilities aimed at improving the quality of care.

20. Two hospitals in the greater Washington, D.C., area began full-scale operations in 1979. This had the effect of driving the total increase in hospital expenses for Maryland in 1979 much higher than it would have been otherwise.

21. J. Graham Atkinson, "Comparison of the Rates of Inflation of Hospitals on Guaranteed Inpatient Revenue Program and Those not on the Program," February 1980 (unpublished).

22. U.S. Department of Health, Education and Welfare, *National Hospital Rate Setting Study, Vol. 6: Case Study of Prospective Reimbursement in New Jersey*, Health Care Financing Grants and Contracts Report, Health Care Financing Administration, April 1980.

23. For a good overview of the historical, conceptual, and technical aspects of the project, see U.S. Department of Health, Education and Welfare, *A Prospective Reimbursement System Based on Patient Case-Mix for New Jersey Hospitals 1976-1983: Third Annual Report, Vol. 1*, Health Care Financing Grants and Contracts Report, Health Care Financing Administration, 15 January 1980.

24. The DRG patient classification system was developed by researchers at Yale University using a newly developed interactive computer system called AUTOGRP; see Robert B. Fetter, et al, "Case Mix Definition by Diagnosis Related Group," *Medical Care* (Supplement), Vol. 18 (February 1980).

25. The Georgia Department of Medical Assistance, under a grant from the Health Care Financing Administration, is conducting an experiment to

develop a DRG-based reimbursement system for medicare and medicaid; the state expects to begin implementing the system for medicaid payments in fall 1980. A case-mix reimbursement study in New York has led to the development of a DRG-based experimental project that is expected to be implemented for several hospitals beginning in early 1981.

26. U.S. Department of Health, Education, and Welfare, *Annual Hospital Report* (Draft for discussion only), Health Care Financing Administration, 20 February 1980.

27. Medicare officials are developing a case-mix feature, using DRGs, to be applied to the system of establishing limits on allowable hospital costs.

6 Health Planning in an Age of Austerity

Louanne Kennedy

Approaches to Planning

The past six years have seen the latest attempt to implement health-planning legislation in the United States. While earlier approaches to health planning were ostensibly aimed at ensuring high-quality medical care to all, since the late 1970s and in 1980 health planning has focused primarily and explicitly on the program of spiraling health-care costs.

The Health Planning and Resources Development Act of 1974 (PL-93-641) provides the institutional framework for an austerity era in health care.[1] The law established a network of state and local health-planning agencies with limited powers to shape local health systems in accordance with nationally established health priorities. The intention was to achieve equal access to quality health care at a reasonable cost: an attempt (on paper at least) to reconcile the expansionist and optimistic activities of the 1960s with the emerging regulatory bent of the 1970s.

PL-93-641 replaced three previous federal programs; Comprehensive Health Planning, the Regional Medical Program, and the Hill-Burton Hospital Construction Program. It created a network of some 205 local Health Systems Agencies (HSAs). HSAs are governed by independent consumer-dominated boards of directors. Elaborate rules govern their composition to assure that they are broadly representative of consumer, provider, and other interests in the community. Each agency is responsible for a health-service area with a population from 500,000 to 3 million, and each has at least one "subarea" or community-level advisory council.[2]

At the state level, the state Health Planning Development Agencies carry out planning, resource allocation, and regulatory functions with the advice of statewide coordinating councils that are governor-appointed bodies similarly representative of the state's population. The state groups roughly parallel the roles and responsibilities of HSAs at the local level.[3]

The development of this multitiered system was to provide both provider and consumer/community input in the planning process. The legislation also emphasized regionalization of services as a major tool of rational planning. A regionalized system is one in which health services are organized at three levels, primary, secondary, and tertiary; corresponding to the incidence of specific types of health needs in the population.

The first five years of the new planning system have been dominated by the contradictions involved in trying to improve health care in an age of austerity when scarcity of resources dominates planning, and yet demands for accessible and accountable personal- and public-health services continue to increase. Two approaches to health planning can be distinguished corresponding to these seemingly contradictory trends: a "system-challenging" approach, and a "system-maintaining" approach.

System-challenging activities challenge the status quo. They may be identified as responding to explicit mandates of the planning legislation to contain costs while at the same time seeking to guarantee accessible, equitable, quality services. System-challenging planning, geared toward improving the health status of the population, finds itself necessarily concerned with restructuring the health system.

System-maintaining planning activities, by contrast, focus on cost containment alone. Existing facilities and patterns of manpower distribution are examined in an effort to reduce potential competition for scarce resources (patients and monies) without basic restructuring of the system. These activities then are geared toward maintenance of the current health-power structure. Such planning typically leads to an emphasis on institutional cutbacks, often disproportionately in the areas of public hospitals and smaller, more fiscally vulnerable community hospitals.

It is suggested here that system-challenging approaches to planning use the current planning legislation. They are dependent on: (1) an HSA board characterized by broad representation of and alliance with consumer groups in the community; (2) an HSA planning methodology that bases assessment of community health needs on population characteristics rather than on needs of existing health institutions and crude resource-to-population measures; (3) aggressive use of HSA certificate-of-need procedures to link planned bed reductions to assured access for communities to both primary preventive care and secondary care as well as to regionally based tertiary services [The cost-containment power of HSAs is in certificate-of-need (CON) reviews. To receive medicaid or medicare reimbursement for the depreciation of any capital expense over $100,000, institutional providers of health care must first receive CON approval.][4]; (4) legal services that assist in identifying the discriminatory aspects of institutional cutbacks as well as broader issues of access for poor and medically indigent populations.

On the other hand, the systems-maintaining approaches to health planning seek to resolve the fiscal pressures on the health system without attacking either the priorities accorded centralized, high-technology care or the assumptions of the medical-engineering model, which have been built into the health-planning effort in the United States since the beginning. Only recently, with austerity, have the full implications of these assumptions become evident.

Health Expenditures

The concern with cost cutting stems ultimately from the rapid increase in expenditures for health care. Between 1974 and 1978, the total amount spent for health care in the United States rose from $115.6 to $192.4 billion (from $501.12 to $820.68 per capita). This increased spending has continued at an undiminished rate.[5]

Growth in health costs has been far more rapid than the growth of the economy as a whole: Health expenditures represented 4.5 percent of the GNP in 1950, 6.2 percent in 1965, 8.8 percent in 1976, and 9.1 percent in 1978. What turned medical inflation into a major concern for national policymakers, however, was not the magnitude or rate of growth in health expenditures but the fact that a large (and growing) proportion of the billions for health came out of public funds. In 1965, 20.3 percent of health-care expenditures came from public funds, in 1978, it was 42 percent of the total.[6]

Thus rising health costs became not merely a matter of individual hardship, as is inflation in other goods and services, but a part of the overall "fiscal crisis of the state." In addition, the rapid rise in health-care expenditures became a matter of concern to large corporations, which found a large and uncontrollably growing portion of their labor costs devoted to health-insurance premiums.

It is the causes and forms of the expenditure crisis, not just its existence in quantitative terms, however, that shape the health-planning response. Changes in population size, population characteristics, or utilization patterns cannot account for the rapid increases in health-care costs. Nor are they a consequence of equal access to medical services by the poor or other groups who for financial reasons were previously excluded from the health-care system.[7]

The increases in expenditures primarily represent the *intensification* of medical care: the increase in the amount of equipment and the number of personnel used per unit of medical service. This is a shift from decentralized, low-technology modes of care to centralized, high-technology modes. These changes are the consequence of third-party cost-reimbursement mechanisms along with the alliance of the medical-supply industries and the large research hospitals that dominate health politics. These institutions recognized early that the more services performed on a patient, the more money would be collected from third-party carriers.

Planning Models and the Politics of Planning

The HSAs were intended to solve the cost problem, but within a system-maintaining framework. Despite this, the new planning mechanism has remained open to some system-planning activites.

Planning is ultimately a political task, not a technical one. Health planning has traditionally depended on resource-based planning—i.e., the use of bed-to-population and similar ratios as the central planning tools for determining issues of over and under bedding. Planners determine regional bed and manpower needs by using formulas incorporating existing utilization data and projected demographic shifts. The use of superficially "value-free" planning techniques seems scientific but is actually inherently biased since it assumes that the current population's use patterns represent necessary utilization levels for appropriate, quality, accessible services. This assumption represents nothing more than the interests of existing health-care institutions; whether it reflects the health needs of the community is open to question.[8]

Consumer- and change-oriented planning requires the use of a new paradigm—population-based planning, which bases its determination of local resource needs on epidemiological studies of the health status and risks on the local population. Politically, this change in "technique" represents a shift away from a planning model that emphasizes the operations and priorities of existing institutions to one that gives priority to the consumers' needs. Indeed, the focus of health-planning ceases to be medical-care institutions per se:

> By basing its analysis on the subsets of the population and their risk levels rather than on the resource structure, population based planning facilitates the identification of the social, economic, and environmental problems which predispose a population to high risk of disease. The methodology, therefore, is capable of addressing an array of health problems that extend well beyond the medical care system, and more adequately accommodates the growing awareness of the social and environmental determinants of health.[9]

Participation of community groups is essential in identifying critical areas of need. Population-based planning identifies the community, rather than the professional, as expert in assessing health requirements. Although the HSA legislation mandates 50 percent consumer membership on boards, consumer-oriented planning can only be assured if those consumer representatives are accountable to organized community-based groups. This is no easy task. Consistent public participation is difficult to achieve since the cost to the citizen is high:

> Participation requires an expenditure of time, effort and money in order to attend hearings, become involved in planning workshops, respond to questionnaires, be interviewed, write letters to officials, secure information about issues, and take part in advisory committees. As these necessary expenditures of resources increase for any particular public decision, an increasing number of citizens are excluded from participation.[10]

The HSA staff can be an invaluable resource in helping consumers participate in health planning. They can play a key role in identifying consumer groups willing and able to assess community needs and generate the political pressure needed to encourage the use of population-based methods rather than the conventional resource-based ones.[11] In addition, staff planners play an important role in ensuring that HSA board membership meets the minimal consumer representation requirement by encouraging information dissemination about HSA activities within the community.[12]

Armed with population-based needs assessments, the CN process, despite its limitations, does provide opportunities for system-challenging activities. For such opportunities to be realized, strong involvement of committed consumer boards is critical. The following list provides examples from across the country of HSAs use of restrictions on CN approvals to increase community access to services and to reduce costly duplicate services.[13]

A California hospital may expand only if it gets another hospital in the area to voluntarily decertify an equal number of beds.

A Western Massachusetts hospital must agree to share new equipment with other hospitals.

A Northern Virginia hospital may acquire equipment only if it switches from proposed lease to a less expensive purchase and passes the savings on in the form of lower charges.

A California Hospital must hire Spanish-speaking staff or sufficient number of translators.

A California nursing home must accept medicaid patients up to 65 percent of its population.

A California nursing home currently spending less money on food (per patient per day) than is spent by the county jail must increase its food budget by 30 percent.

A Western Masschusetts HMO must agree to sliding scale based on ability to pay.

A North Central Georgia hospital may expand only if it provides $150,000 for care of indigents. (This compromise was reached shortly after the local HSA reorganized its board to give greater consumer representation and accountability—a response to the October 1979 federal legislation.)

A recent California case provides an example of some of the dynamics involved in such uses of the CON level: The Scripps Institute in LaJolla,

California, requested approval for an $8 million expansion program. In its application, Scripps argued that it served the entire community. HSA staff and community board members uncovered data that showed that 17 percent of the population in the LaJolla area were eligible for medicaid, while patient profiles at Scripps showed that only 1.8 percent of Scripps patients were medicaid recipients. With the community able to argue persuasively that access to the facility by medicaid patients could not be demonstrated, the application was turned down at the board level. Ultimately, in order to gain approval for its plan, Scripps agreed to provide $300,000 for the local Council of Community Clinics and to guarantee it would donate all its used medical equipment to the clinics.[14]

While these decisions may seem minor victories in the face of continued expansion of medical empires, they do demonstrate the HSA's potential to improve local health services.

Hospital Closings and Issues of Access to Care

The examples cited are of the use of planning mechanisms to force improvements in the accessibility, quality, or efficiency of health services. Unfortunately, the most pressing health-planning issue in the present period of austerity is the maintenance of already minimal service threatened with extinction. Here legal strategies (often spearheaded by the National Health Law Program, the Consumer Coalition for Health, and various local Neighborhood Legal Services Groups) have been central, although they too require relevant population-based data.

The recent wave of hospital closings has affected both medicaid recipients and the medically indigent.

> The medically indigent population, which is highly dependent on public hospitals, encompasses many persons not classified as poor according to traditional measures of poverty. Substantial numbers of people are ineligible for federal and state programs, and lack private health insurance, yet are unable to pay for necessary medical care.[15]

Public hospitals have traditionally been the source of care of last resort for this group. Cost-containment legislation and mounting fiscal pressures across the nation on state and local governments have led to forced closures of public hospitals. Counting on private hospitals to pick up the slack, cities such as New York, Detroit, St. Louis, and Philadelphia operate on what Quentin Young, Cook County Hospital Medical Director, has called the "Marie Antoinette" theory of health-care reform. This is the belief that the poor, no longer able to receive care at public hospitals, will now be welcomed by the private hospitals that have spurned them for so long.

But it is not only the public hospitals that are being closed to solve the fiscal crisis. Unable, or unwilling, to constrain the massive amount of unnecessary hospitalization and surgery for which the government pays, the federal Health Care Financing Administration is seeking to control its budget by constricting the amount of reimbursement available to hospitals and private physicians who treat medicaid beneficiaries. These policies have forced many private hospitals into financial crisis. They now face bankruptcy not because of mismanagement or drastic overbuilding or lack of need for their services, but from their unwillingness to close their doors to the poor. Of the twenty-four private hospitals that closed in New York City between 1974 and 1978, 85 percent were in or on the border of medically underserved poverty communities.[16]

The conventional justification for such closings is the high cost of maintaining excess bed capacity. No one questions that overbedding exists. The crisis is over *which* underused hospitals will be designated for service reductions or closure. Alan Sager has shown that:

> Closings and relocations (to suburban, more financially secure areas) appear to have been disproportionately by certain types of hospitals located disproportionately in certain types of neighborhoods. . . . As the minority proportion of the neighborhood around the hospital increases so does the proportion of hospitals closing or relocating. . . . In neighborhoods which were less than 25 percent black in 1970, for example, only 14.2 percent of the 1937 hospitals had closed or relocated by 1977. But in neighborhoods which were more than 3/4 black in 1970, fully 46.9 percent of hospitals—almost half—had disappeared.[17]

My own studies suggest that excess hospital capacity per se is not highly correlated with which hospitals are singled out for closing. The single strongest predictive variable for urban areas is the percentage of minority population in the surrounding area. For all areas of three states studied over nineteen years, it is predominantly the small low-cost hospitals in rural and urban areas that are singled out for closure.[18] Studies such as these give credence to the activists' conclusion that the official concern with overbedding is in reality a smokescreen for the real issue of maintaining profits and power for a few institutions and cutting costs in the rest.

As the process continues and smaller hospitals providing primary and secondary care in both rural and urban areas continue to be driven toward bankruptcy and closure, we are faced with the clear possibility of having to reinvent the community hospital. The intent of PL-93-641 to regionalize services (that is, to coordinate and rationalize resources for primary, secondary, and tertiary care within appropriate geographical boundaries) is subverted by the process of cost containment. The surviving institutions are disproportionately the medical empires—large expensive tertiary-care-oriented hospitals able to maintain high occupancy rates but also exhibiting the highest cost per patient day.[19]

The single most important focus for consumer-oriented planners at the present time is the struggle against the racially and economically discriminatory, and grotesquely uneconomical, patterns of hospital closings. Success in such struggles requires coordinated action by community groups, legal services, and Health Systems Agencies.

Agency and community activists in New York, California, Illinois, and elsewhere have united around such struggles, although with limited success. Examples of effective health-planning activity leading to substantially increased access to quality health services have been hard to come by in recent years. In an age when merely preventing already inadequate services from deteriorating further is seen as a victory, it is tempting to be cynical about the entire health-planning process.

It is evident, however, that those responsible for cutbacks see the existing health-planning system as a significant obstacle. The federal government appears to be moving toward the abolition of locally based Health Systems Agencies, replacing them with state- and federal-level planning agencies that would presumably be less sensitive to community pressures (that is, perceived community needs). Such a change would remove the last barriers to a wholesale assault on health services for minorities and the poor. On the positive side, health planning based in local areas has encouraged a broader view of health, not focused solely on current legislation and existing institutions but including issues of workplace health, school health, and environmental health.

The struggle for planners oriented toward the "system-challenging" approach in the 1980s, then, lies in two areas. First, they must respond to the pressures for cost reduction by designing bed reductions and other changes in existing institutions and reimbursement mechanisms that increase the efficiency and effectiveness of the health system while not adversely affecting the poor's access to services. And second, they must maintain their commitment to locally based planning agencies with mechanisms for strong community input and accountability to the community.

Notes

1. 41 (No. 60) *Federal Register* (Friday, 26 March 1976, Sec. 122).

2. Of the local HSAs formed, about three fourths have final designation by HEW, and most of the rest are at least conditionally designated. Consumers comprise 53 percent of all HSA board members. Boards vary in size from a low of 15 to a high of 137. Subarea advisory councils, covering the community or local area of planning, vary in number from Arizona Area I with a single council composed of 15 members to New York Area VII in New York City having 33 councils. Total board membership across the country numbers 15,000.

3. For further discussion of the National Health Planning and Resources Development Act of 1974, see, for example, Steven Sieverts, *Health Planning Issues and Public Law 93-641* (Blue Cross Association, 1977).

4. Herbert Hyman, *Regulating Health Facilities Construction* (Aspen Systems, 1977). See also David Abernethy and David Pearson, *Regulating Hospital Costs: The Development of Public Policy* (AUPHA Press, 1979).

5. *Statistical Abstract of the United States, 1979*, pp. 100-101.

6. Ibid.

7. Lynn Naliboff and Dorothy Lang, "Expanding Access to Health Care: Written Eligibility Standards for the Medically Indigent," *Clearinghouse Review*: 849:

> Restrictions and inconsistencies in Medicaid eligibility standards are such that in 1974, 9.5 million persons with incomes below the poverty line, or 39 percent of that population were not covered by Medicaid. In 1975 the proportion of the poor and near poor ineligible for Medicaid or Medicare reached 62 percent in South Dakota and 66 percent in Mississippi. Thus, while legislation acknowledges that there exists a medically needy population not poor enough to qualify for welfare, in practice not even the narrowly defined poverty population receives adequate medical coverage.

Since 1965 the government has assumed financial responsibility for paying for care for large numbers of the poor. But while this factor may explain some of the health-expenditure increases of the 1960s, it has little to do with the sustained increases since then.

8. See Louis Tannen, "Health Planning as a Regulatory Strategy: A Discussion of History and Current Uses," *International Journal of Health Services* (Winter 1979).

9. Ibid.

10. Theodore Marmor and James Morone, "HSAs and the Representation of Consumer Interests: Conceptual Issues and Litigation Problems," *Health Law Project Library Bulletin* 4 (April 1979):117-128. See also Bruce Vladeck, "Interest Group Representation and the HSAs: Health Planning and Political Theory," *American Journal of Public Health* 67 (January 1977):23-29.

11. Barry Checkoway and Michael Doyle, "Community Organizing Lessons for Health Care Consumers," *Journal of Health Politics, Policy and Law* (May/ June, 1979).

12. Ibid. See Also John Bradley, "Volunteer Education: Key to Building an Effective Planning Process," *Health Law Project Library Bulletin* 4 (May 1979): 164-172.

13. The range of certificate-of-needs experiences is drawn from personal correspondence with Mark Kleiman, Consumer Coalition for Health, Washington, D.C., and from the CHAM newsletter published by the coalition. The range of experience around CON was summarized by Kleiman for use by congressional staff.

14. Ibid.

15. Naliboff and Lang, "Expanding Access to Health Care," p. 848.

16. Proceedings of the Health Policy Forum, "Hospital Closures in New York City," No. 2, United Hospital Fund, February 1980.

17. Alan Sager, "Urban Hospital Closings in the Face of Racial Change, a Statement on Hospital Financing Problems," testimony before the Subcommittee on Health, Committee on Ways and Means, U.S. House of Representatives, 14 March 1980.

18. Louanne Kennedy, "Comparing Closures, Survivors and New Hospitals in Three States," Conference on Fighting for the Public Hospital, Maryland, May 1980.

19. Louanne Kennedy and Barbara Caress, "A Longitudinal Analysis of Hospital Behavior in Three States: 1960-1979," unpublished manuscript.

7

Physicians' Assistants as Innovative Health-Care-Delivery Mechanisms

James L. Regens and
Mark R. Daniels

During the past decade, the health-care industry has made tremendous efforts to supply manpower to meet the spiraling health needs of a rapidly growing population. Faced with predicted reports of huge personnel shortages from the 1960s on into the 1980s, the immediate response has been to produce more doctors, nurses, and dentists as well as paraprofessional personnel trained in techniques that mirrored the skills of professionals. Of prime concern was the anticipated shortage of physicians. Increasing the number of physicians in this country, however, is a lengthy process. For example, physicians are required to take a year of internship after medical school before assuming a practice, and most take a two- to four-year residency. This produces a relatively long lag time between the start of medical training and actual independent practice.

Physicians' assistants (PAs) were conceived as an innovative health-care-delivery mechanism that would help to alleviate the doctor shortage. Although receiving much less training than physicians over a shorter time span, they would be capable of performing certain tasks that would save the physician time and effort. Consequently, the title "physician's assistant" is a generic term referring to health-care practitioners who perform tasks ordinarily reserved for a physician. They commonly assist, under the direction of a physician, in the diagnostic and therapeutic management of patients.[1] Supporters assert that widespread utilization of PAs would affect health-care delivery in several of ways. First, they could offer primary care in a limited form where medical manpower is unavailable or inaccessible. Second, they potentially increase the efficiency and productivity of the individual physician by assuming simple and repetitive tasks associated with his or her practice so that the physician can see more patients.[2]

State Authorization of Physicians' Assistants

Historically the idea of using such midlevel health practitioners to supplement physicians can be traced to 1965 when a two-year training program was instituted at Duke University. Soon thereafter, the Stanford University Medical

Center established a two-year PAs program, Aderson-Broadduss College started a four-year college-based program, and the University of Colorado began a five-year Child Health Associate program designed to train assistants for pediatricians. By 1972 twenty-one of the thirty-one programs in operation were supported by federal agencies while the remainder were financed by private foundations and institutional sources. However, the amount of federal revenues allocated for these programs is relatively small (for example, only $35 million for fiscal year 1979).[3] As a result, the primary impact of federal funds has been to help existing rather than new programs. Overall, the total number of programs has remained fairly constant. From 1972 to 1977, ten new programs were started and eight programs closed.[4] As of 1977, there were thirty-three programs located in 29 states.[5] Reasons for closing have varied, but for the most part they have involved economic support problems, graduate-placement difficulties, and lack of support for PAs from other health-care providers.[6] Nonetheless, as of January 1979, 44 states have adopted legislation that permits PAs certification under either regulatory or delagatory guidelines. In order to better understand the factors underlying state legislatures' willingness to experiment with such a nontraditional approach to providing medical services, this research identifies the extent and explores the conditions under which states are willing to authorize the adoption of this relatively new health-care-delivery mechanism.

Certifying Physicians' Assistants

The general purpose of professional licensing is to protect the public from fraud and incompetence by ensuring that a licensed practioner possesses some minimum acceptable level of training and skills.[7] For paraprofessional occupations such as physicians' assistants, certification of individuals who met certain set standards represents a regulatory alternative to licensing. Since the certification process is less restrictive and normally applies to occupations instead of professions, it occasionally is referred to as "permissive licensing."[8] Consequently, in the health-care area, because PAs work under licensed physicians, they are usually certified by state regulatory agencies.[9]

In order to have a current assessment of the number of states that have adopted PAs legislation, a survey of the 50 states was conducted during the first three months of 1979. A combination of mailed questionnaires and telephone interviews were directed to the board of medical examiners or in its absence, the appropriate state agency. Table 7-1 reveals that as of January 1979, 44 states have enacted certification legislation permitting PAs to practice under the direction, supervision, and responsibility of a licensed physician.[10] No state that has adopted legislation authorizing PAs has subsequently repealed it. Moreover, no regional patterns of adoption are apparent.

Table 7-1
Incidence and Variation of PAs Policy Formulation by State

State	Year	Regulatory	Delegatory	Number of Prohibited Activities[b]	Physician Supervision[c]
Alabama	1971	X		1	1
Alaska	1974	X		4	1
Arizona	1972	X		4	1
Arkansas	1977	X		4	2
California	1975	X		2	3
Colorado	[a]			2	4
Connecticut	1971		X	2	4
Delaware	1971		X	1	4
Florida	1971	X		4	2
Georgia	1972	X		3	3
Hawaii	1973		X	1	1
Idaho	1972	X		3	1
Illinois	1976	X		3	3
Indiana	1977	X		2	4
Iowa	1971	X		1	3
Kansas	1978	X		4	4
Kentucky				4	4
Louisiana	1977	X		2	3
Maine	1973	X		4	3
Maryland	1973	X		1	4
Massachusetts	1973	X		3	4
Michigan	1977	X		1	2
Minnesota	1978	X		4	4
Mississippi				4	4
Missouri				4	4
Montana				4	4
Nebraska	1973	X		3	3
Nevada	1973	X		3	2
New Hampshire	1971	X		1	2
New Jersey				4	4
New Mexico	1973	X		3	2
New York	1972	X		3	3
North Carolina	1971	X		1	4
North Dakota	1975	X		3	1
Ohio	1976	X		3	2
Oklahoma	1972	X		1	2
Oregon	1971	X		3	2
Pennsylvania	1978	X		2	4
Rhode Island	1976	X		3	3
South Carolina	1974	X		3	2
South Dakota	1974	X		3	2
Tennessee	1973		X	1	4
Texas	1975	X		3	3
Utah	1971	X		4	4
Vermont	1971	X		4	1
Virginia	1973	X		1	2
Washington	1971	X		3	1
West Virginia	1976	X		3	3

Table 7-1 — *(Continued)*

State	Year	Regulatory	Delegatory	Number of Prohibited Activities[b]	Physician Supervision[c]
Wisconsin	1973	X		4	2
Wyoming	1973	X		1	1

[a]Only child-health associate.

[b]Prohibited activites by states that have PAs certification legislation include: optometry, dentistry, pharmacy, independent judgment, chiropractic, hearing aids, nursing, operative treatment, fracture treatment, podiatry, psychology. Numerical codes are: 1 = single prohibited activity; 2 = two prohibited activities; 3 = three or more prohibited activities; 4 = none or not stated.

[c]Numerical codes are: 1 = under supervision of physician; 2 = availability of physician; 3 = review by physician; 4 = regulations or not stated.

Some states do not specify in their statute or regulations what functions may not be performed by PAs. Presumably, in those states lacking prohibited activities, physicians' assistants may perform whatever tasks are authorized by their supervising physicians. On the other hand, in many states, PAs are prohibited from performing certain activities. For example, Indiana and several other states prohibit PAs from performing independent diagnosis, treatment, or prescription without consultation with a physician.[11] Georgia specifically prohibits a physicians' assistant from performing any tasks not listed on the job description submitted to the regulatory agency.[12] New Mexico, South Carolina, and Ohio have a long list of specifically prohibited medical tasks.[13] In fact, most PA regulatory statutes explicitly prohibit performing medical procedures except under the supervision of a physician. Although the states are not in unanimous agreement on the degree of physician supervision that should be maintained, no state requires the physical presence of the physician while the PA is performing services, either in the same room or even at the same facility.[14]

Identifying the Determinants of State Authorization

State legislatures face three possible policy choices regarding the formulation of PAs legislation. The first policy choice is whether or not to permit the use of physicians' assistants. Those states that allow PAs to work in the health field then face a second policy choice: whether to adopt a general delegatory or a regulatory statute.[15] General delegatory statutes involve an amendment to the state's medical-practice act giving physicians authority to use PAs at their discretion. The regulatory approach gives an organization, usually the state board of medical examiners, authority to establish rules and regulations pertaining to the education and practice of PAs. Variation among the states in the adoption as well as content of legislation enabling PAs to provide health services leads to two policy-related questions. First, what factors are associated with variation among the states in their willingness to adopt PAs legislation? Second, what factors are associated with variation in the type of enabling legislation that is adopted? In order to answer these questions, we now examine the degree to which theoretically relevant state characteristics affect those policy choices.

Health-Care Demand

As mentioned earlier, physicians' assistants commonly offer primary health services in areas where medical manpower is unavailable or inaccessible. They also frequently allow doctors to see more patients by assuming simple and repetitive tasks otherwise normally performed by a physician. Consequently, PAs may greatly aid in the delivery of health-care services, especially in states where health-care demand is high.

Numerous studies suggest that only a few variables exhibit a strong role in explaining the demand for health care.[16] For example, price appears to account for a relatively small percentage of the variation in demand.[17] Nonetheless, when services are free, demand does rise significantly, which suggests that health-care expenditures increase as consumer income increases.[18] Other research finds that health-care demand differs with age, sex, birthrates, and marital status.[19] Specifically the number of physician visits is higher for the young (under five years), the old (sixty-five and over), and for women in child-bearing ages. Marital status also affects demand because a single person living alone may seek hospital care for an illness that would require care only at home for a person living with his or her family.[20]

Socioeconomic Conditions

Measures of social and economic conditions have been identified as frequent determinants of state policy choices.[21] As noted previously, affluence may affect the demand for health care both in terms of the frequency with which individuals avail themselves of services as well as the sophistication of the technology employed to deliver those services. Similarly, cultural characteristics may also influence health-care demand.[22] In order to test the hypothesis that socioeconomic conditions do in fact influence state PAs legislation, our analysis includes indicators of affluence and industrialization.[23]

Medical-Community Reaction

The use of PAs as an alternative to physicians in providing certain health-care services is controversial within the health professions. A variety of professional associations have spoken out concerning the status of PAs legislation. Some states, for example, have experienced bitter lobbying against the adoption of such legislation because of opposition from state medical associations.[24] In fact, opinion about PAs is evenly divided among private, general-practice physicians. In a recent national survey of physicians, only 51 percent of non-group, general-practice physicians approved of "non-MD associates" who work "independently to some extent in underdoctored areas."[25] Much of the opposition of PAs appears to come from rural general or family practitioners.[26] Presumably, these physicians feel that their earnings or prestige may be undermined when PAs perform medical duties previously provided by licensed physicians. As a result, because a major task of a professional association is to maintain as much influence as possible over admission standards to and competition with the profession, this may mean that state medical associations attempt to greatly influence the substance of the PAs statute by consulting with state legislators or by actually writing the statute for the state legislature. It may also mean, of course, determined opposition to any type of PAs statute. Consequently, the salience of PAs as a controversial issue confronting physicians and the relative size, strength, and position of state medical associations are variables that may have an effect on PAs policy formulation.[27]

Policy Innovativeness

State policy choices have also been found to be influenced by the general tendency of state governments to intervene in new policy areas. For example, Walker maintains that the speed of adoption of different social policies is realtively constant for any particular state.[28] Presumably, the overall willingness of a state to experiment with other new policy approaches may affect its willingness to authorize the use of PAs as a health-care delivery mechanism.[29]

Discriminant analysis provides an appropriate statistical technique for predicting state adoption of PAs legislation as well as the type of enabling legislation adopted based on the preceding structural characteristics. In this research a single function representing a linear combination of the set of independent variables that distinguishes one choice from another for both of the policy options is produced. The standardized coefficients for the independent variables measure their relative predictive capability. They are similar in interpretation to beta weights while the eta^2 coefficient is comparable to the R^2 value in regression analysis. Interpretation of the sign for each independent variable on the discriminant functions is keyed to the sign of the group centroids for the function. The group centroids are the mean values for each category of the scores that serve as an index to classify each case into the most appropriate category of the dependent variable.[30]

Table 7-2 identifies which characteristics best discriminate adopting from nonadopting states. For this portion of our analysis, a positive sign on the centroids, and thus for the independent variables on the discriminant function, is related to adoption of PAs legislation. Clearly, as a group, the indicators of the medical community's reaction—especially the lobbying strength of the state medical association—are the most discriminating predictors. Socioeconomic conditions are also strongly related to the willingness of states to authorize the use of physicians' assistants in the health-services area. On the other hand, while the birth rate does appear to affect the adoption of PAs legislation, our other measure of health-care demand plays a relatively insignificant role. The general willingness of a state to adopt new policies also appears to exert only a minor influence on the adoption of this specific innovation. The analysis succeeds in classifying correctly state legislative decisions for a large percentage of the cases (87.2 percent), with moderate overall predictive capability.[31]

In addition to examining the characteristics underlying state authorization of the use of physicians' assistants, our analysis also explores why states adopt regulatory as opposed to delegatory statutes. Table 7-3 reveals that, just as the medical community's reaction influences whether or not a state permits PAs to provide health-care services, it also affects the type of enabling legislation

Table 7-2
Discriminant Analysis of State Adoption of PAs Legislation

Groups	*Group Centroids*
Adopters	0.260
Nonadopters	−2.182

	Standardized Discriminant-Function Coefficients
Health-care demand	
Young women, children	.130
Birthrate	.888
Socioeconomic conditions	
Affluence	.783
Industrialization	.865
Medical-community reaction	
State medical-association support	.861
State medical-association lobbying strength	−.907
Symbolic significance	−.835
Policy innovativeness	
General innovativeness score	−.320
Predictive capability = 87.2%	Eta^2 = .372

Table 7-3

Discriminant Analysis of State Adoption of Delegatory and Regulatory PAs Legislation

Groups	Group Centroids
Delegatory	−2.319
Regulatory	0.178

Health-care demand	Standardized Discriminant-Function Coefficients
Young women, children	.026
Birthrate	.280
Socioeconomic conditions	
Affluence	.015
Industrialization	−.615
Medical-community reaction	
State medical-association support	.439
State medical-association lobbying strength	.687
Symbolic significance	−.155
Policy innovativeness	
General innovativeness	−.012
Predictive capability = 88.1%	Eta^2 = .272

adopted. Regulatory statutes that are generally more restrictive are more likely to result if the state medical association supports the use of PAs but also has strong lobbying capabilities.[32] However, once a state decides to permit PAs to deliver health-care services, the issue's symbolic salience diminishes and has little impact on the type of statute adopted. Furthermore, general policy innovativeness and health-care demand both exert only a marginal effect on statutory content.

Conclusion

Physicians' assistants represent a new health-care-delivery mechanism designed to supply additional manpower and cope with the spiraling demands for health care. Most states have enacted regulatory legislation that permits PAs to practice within their boundaries. In addition, over half of the states have training programs for PAs, supported in part by the federal government.

While PAs legislation is meant to improve health-care delivery by creating a new cadre of medical personnel, our findings indicate that variation in the level of state health-care demand is not an important determinant of what legislative policy choices states actually make regarding the use of PAs as an approach to providing health-care services. In fact, our study reveals that the most important predictor of state legislative decisions on new approaches to the staffing of medical services may be the extent to which the medical associations is related to the passage of PAs legislation, while the relative lobbying strength of those associations is linked to adoption of a regulatory statute. As mentioned earlier, a major task of a professional association is to maintain as much influence as is possible over standards of admission to the profession. Thus in order for state medical associations to affect the standards of admission to the closely related occupation of PAs, it appears necessary for them to support the legislation authorizing such an approach to health-care delivery. Moreover, if its lobbying abilities are well established, a state medical association may influence the substance of the statute by consulting with legislators or by actually writing the legislation. Such support and consultation generally results in nondiscretionary, regulatory statutes. As a result, by supporting PAs legislation, a state medical association with a well-established lobby protects the interests of its members by increasing the likelihood of obtaining a regulatory statute that establishes rules and regulations governing the education and practices of PAs.

Because this study examines the adoption of a relatively new health-care-delivery mechanism, its findings form the basis for enhanced understanding of the conditions under which states are willing to experiment with nontraditional approaches to providing medical services. In this respect, health policymakers should be aware that an interest group's perception of how its membership may be affected by a new health policy may be a more important determinant of the policy decisions that state legislatures make than are actual levels of state health-care demand.

Notes

1. Association of Physician Assistant Programs, *National Health Practitioner Program Profile, 1979-1980* (Arlington, Va.: Author, 1978).

2. David Mechanic, "Politics, Social Scence and Health Policy in the U.S.," in David Mechanic, ed., *Politics, Medicine and Social Science* (New York: Wiley, 1974).

3. This federal support represented an investment in experimental programs to test the hypothesis that midlevel health professionals could provide many physician-equivalent services in primary and continuing care.

4. A. Bliss and E. Cohen, *The New Health Professionals: Nurse Practitioners and Physicians' Assistants* (Germantown, Md.: Aspen Systems Corporation, 1977).

5. The following states have PA training programs: Alaska, California, Connecticut, Florida, Georgia, Iowa, Kansas, Maryland, Massachusetts, Michigan, Missouri, Nebraska, Nevada, New Hampshire, New Jersey, New Mexico, New York, North Carolina, North Dakota, Ohio, Oklahoma, Pennsylvania, South Carolina, Tennessee, Texas, Utah, Washington, West Virginia, and Wisconsin.

6. Bliss and Cohen, *The New Health Professionals.*

7. H. Goldstein and M. Horowitz, *Entry-Level Health Occupations: Development and Future* (Baltimore, Md.: Johns Hopkins University Press, 1977).

8. Ibid.

9. Personal communication, Robert Curry, Director of the Physicians' Assistants Program, Emory University School of Medicine, February 1979.

10. Colorado has a statute regulating "child health associates." Although some studies have considered these associates to be PAs, the Colorado Board of Medical Examiners denied that they have a PAs statute when surveyed in connection with this study. For further information on Colorado's statute, see Department of Health, Education and Welfare, *Review and Analysis of State Legislation and Reimbursement Practices of Physicians' Assistants and Nurse Practitioners: Final Report* (Washington, D.C.: Author, 1978). Therefore, for purposes of this study, we treat Colorado as a nonadopter.

11. Indiana Code 25-22. 5-1-1(i).

12. Georgia Code Annotated 84-62.

13. See New Mexico Statutes Annotated 67-5-3.1; Code of Laws of South Carolina, 40-47-69(4); Ohio Regulatory Codes, Chapter 4730.

14. Department of Health, Education and Welfare, *Review and Analysis.*

15. Ibid.

16. See P.J. Feldstein, "The Demand for Medical Care," in The Commission on the Cost of Medical Care, ed., *General Report* Vol. 1 (Chicago: American Medical Association, 1964); P.J. Feldstein and J.W. Carr, "The Effect of Income on Medical Care Spending," in American Statistical Association, *Proceedings of the Social Sciences Section* (Washington, D.C.: Author, 1964); G.D. Rosenthal, *The Demand for General Hospital Facilities* (Chicago: American Hospital Association, 1964); M.S. Feldstein, *Economic Analysis for Health Science Efficiency* (Amsterdam, Netherlands: North Holland Publishing Company, 1967); S.G. Long, Demand for Medical Care (Unpublished doctoral dissertation, University of Iowa, 1969); C. Stewart and C. Siddayao, *Increasing the Supply of Medical Personnel* (Washington, D.C.: American Enterprise Institute for Public Policy Research, 1973); M. Cooper, *Rationing Health Care* (New York: Wiley, 1975); L. Weeks and H. Berman, eds., *Economics in Health Care* (Germantown, Md.: Aspen Systems Corporation, 1977). A.J. Culyer and K.G. Wright, *Economic Aspects of Health Services* (London: Robertson and Company, 1978); T.L. Hall and A. Mejia, *Health Manpower Planning* (Geneva, Switzerland: World Health Organization, 1978).

17. Weeks and Berman, *Economics in Health Care.*

18. In this study, affluence is included as a distinct independent variable.

19. Stewart and Siddayao, *Increasing the Supply of Medical Personnel.*

20. The health-care demand variables included in this study are based on age, sex, birthrates, and marital status. The two measures of age are the

percentage of individuals under five years of age and over sixty-five years of age relative to the total population of a state. Sex is measured by the percentage of women in childbearing ages relative to the total female population of a state, and the birthrate of a state is measured by the number of children born per 1000 women ever married aged fifteen to forty-four. The indicator of birthrate is not so much a measure of how many infants there are in a state but rather of the relative rate of births per 1000 women. Marital status is the percentage of single individuals not including those separated, widowed, or divorced, over fourteen years of age relative to the total population of a state. Factor analysis performed on the health-care-demand variables with the exception of the birthrate variable produces one dimension, named Young Women/ Children. All data for the health demand variables are collected from the United States Bureau of the Census, Census of Population, 1970.

21. For a review of this literature, see M.S. Lewis-Beck, "The Relative Importance of Socioeconomic and Political Variables for Public Policy," *American Political Science Review* 71 (June 1977):559-566.

22. Examples of the relationship between cultural characteristics and health-care demand include: states with high proportions of Scandinavians have low rates of demand, and nonwhites tend to have higher levels of demand for health care than do whites. See Stewart and Siddayao, *Increasing the Supply of Medical Personnel.*

23. Data for the affluence and industrialization levels for each state were measured using factor scores taken from D.R. Morgan and W. Lyons, "Industrialization and Affluence Revisited: A Note on Socioeconomic Dimensions of the American States," *American Journal of Political Science* 40 (May 1975): 263-276.

24. For example, the Pharmacy Association of Georgia, the Nursing Association of Georgia, and the Georgia Medical Association have all lobbied for a resolution rescinding PAs certification legislation. See Curry, personal communication.

25. David Mechanic, "Policy Studies and Medical Care Research," in David Mechanic, ed., *Politics, Medicine and Social Science* (New York: Wiley, 1974).

26. Curry, personal communication.

27. For a discussion of the characteristics that explain the variations in the role and effectiveness of interest groups, see J.Q. Wilson, *Political Organizations* (New York: Basic Books, 1973), pp. 303-310. The characteristics of state medical associations chosen for analysis are: (1) the position of the state medical association in terms of no action, or the adoption of a formal resolution supporting or opposing PAs; (2) the size of the state medical association staff relative to the total membership; (3) whether it has a full- or part-time lobbyist; (4) whether or not the lobbyist has a full-time office in the state capitol; and (5) the relative number of rural general/family practitioners as a measure of salience. Factor analysis performed on the political variables with the exception

of the salience variable produces two dimensions, named Support and Lobbying Strength. A telephone survey of all fifty state medical associations was conducted during the spring of 1979 in order to collect the data for the variables. An attempt was made to interview the executive director of each medical association. If this was not possible, a lobbyist or legislative researcher for the state medical association was interviewed. Questionnaires were completed for all states except Mississippi and Alaska. Data for the salience variable was collected from the U.S. Bureau of Census, Census of Population, 1970.

28. J.L. Walker, "The Diffusion of Innovations Among the American States," *American Political Science Review* 63 (September 1969):880-899.

29. An index that measures the adoption rate of 69 new policies across the entire array of state functions (for example, health, environment, social welfare, business regulation, and criminal justice) during the period 1930-1970 was employed in this study to assess the relative level of general policy innovativeness for each state, see R. Savage, "Policy Innovativeness as a Trait of American States," *Journal of Politics* 40 (February 1978):212-224.

30. Although regression and discriminant produce standardized coefficients that can be interpreted in the same fashion, the two techniques have distinct theoretical objectives. Regression focuses on minimizing error terms to predict variance for an interval dependent variable. Discriminant maximizes category (group) separation to establish values for the functions that will classify each case in the most appropriate category of a non-interval-dependent variable. In discriminant models, the number of functions is equal to the number of categories in the dependent variable minus one or the number of independent variables minus one, whichever is less. For additional discussion, see W.W. Cooley and P.R. Lohnes, *Multivariate Data Analysis* (New York: Wiley, 1971).

31. In discriminant analysis, a priori and a posteriori probabilities of group membership should be compared. By classifying cases to the modal group in each analysis, the mean a priori predictive capability equals 91.1 percent. Using the discriminant function for each analysis to classify cases produces a mean a posteriori predictive capability of 87.7 percent. The mean predictive capability of the discriminant functions is essentially equivalent to the mean predictive capability of the modal classification. For further discussion about evaluating the predictive power of discriminant analyses, see Cooley and Lohnes, *Multivariate Data Analysis.*

32. For table 7-3, a positive sign is related to the passage of a regulatory statute.

Part IV
Financing

8

Planning for National Health Insurance by Objective: The Contract Mechanism

Steven Jonas

Introduction

National health insurance (NHI) has been on the national political agenda of the United States since 1912 when Teddy Roosevelt included an NHI plank in the platform of his Bull Moose Party. Most consideration of national-health-insurance proposals are more recently, proposals for a national health service (NHS), begin from one of the following premises:

1. NHI/NHS is morally good because it is equitable; therefore, the United States ought to have it.
2. NHI/NHS is bad because it would mean "government interference" and "skyrocketing costs"; anyway it isn't needed. If there is to be a plan, it must be designed so that it causes the least change in the status quo and the least harm to identified self-interests.
3. NHI/NHS is a political subject. In one form or another, a plan might be politically helpful to its proposer. Therefore a plan should be developed.

In premises such as these, assessments of the needs of the American people for health services do not receive much consideration or evaluation. Rather, it is moral values, self-interest, or political considerations that are given most weight. Since needs, goals, and health-related program objectives do not come first, NHI/NHS plans that are developed on one of these premises often begin with, and sometimes never get beyond, being designed to meet *process* rather than *outcome* objectives. Thus a great deal of time can be spent on issues such as "government interference," "community control," copayment, the preservation or end of private practice, the inclusion or elimination of private insurance companies, and the preservation or end of the voluntary hospital as we know it.

The approach to NHI outlined herein begins with a different premise. Data clearly demonstrate that the health status of the American people is not as good as it could be, assuming that existing knowledge and techniques for health promotion and disease prevention and treatment were fully implemented [1]. Furthermore, data clearly indicate that some of the present features of the U.S. health-care-delivery system inhibit the development of a system that would be more beneficial for the health of the American people than the present one is [2]. The assumption is made that improved health status is a desirable goal for several reasons: The changes of survival of the species and its American subset will be improved, productivity will be improved, money will be saved, and people will be happier. It should be noted that morality plays a minor role in this rationale. Thus this approach to development of an NHI plan begins with a needs assessment.

Needs Assessment for National-Health-Insurance Planning

Health Status

The American people bear an unnecessary burden of at least partially preventable disease and disability. The top killers—heart disease, cancer, stroke, accidents, diabetes, cirrhosis of the liver, influenza and pneumonia, bronchitis and emphysema, and suicide—are all amenable to at least partial reduction in their severity as causes of death an disability by known preventive measures [1]. Certain common usually nonfatal causes of disability are also susceptible to reduction by known preventive measures: venereal disease, tuberculosis, occupational and environmental exposures to harmful substances, measles, and obesity. Beyond a concern for specific diseases and their prevention, health itself as a positive state can be promoted. It is now well known that proper nutrition, exercise, avoidance of cigarettes, a reasonable amount of exercise, moderation in alcohol consumption, and stress management can improve health not just in terms of reducing the risks of getting specific diseases but also in the positive sense of feeling better and functioning more effectively [3]. Finally, although all American citizens could benefit from being provided with the opportunity to lead healthier lives if they chose to do so, there are certain groups in the population that are clearly less healthy than the national average [4]. They could benefit from special programs.

Medical-Care Issues

There are a number of problems with the system for delivering medical care (treatment) services that are well known [2]. Unless the current (1979-1980) sag in the rate of medical-care-cost increase is not an unusual, probably artefactual situation, the most serious problem facing the medical-care-delivery system is the rapid rise in costs. Health services as a whole consume about 9 percent of the gross national product [5]. This is up from 5.3 percent in 1960. There are serious concerns with the quality of medical care [6]. The geographic and specialty maldistribution of personnel and facilities is well known. This creates major problems in access to care in certain parts of the country. There are organizational and administrative inefficiencies and fragmentation of services [7]. Finally, there are some serious problems in doctor-patient communication [8] and with the role of health and patient education in the system [9].

Provider Concerns

There are two groups of people in any health-care-delivery system: the patients and the providers. (To some, "providers" is a pejorative term; I do not intend it to be pejorative. It is all encompassing, covering professional and nonprofessional healthworkers.) Providers have needs too. Just as in NHI design, patient needs must be taken into account from the beginning in planning, so too must provider needs. For one reason or another, it may be neither feasible nor desirable to meet all identified provider needs. (The same applies to patient needs too.) But they should be recognized, evaluated, and given priorities. The providers include: physicians and other fee-for-service providers, salaried healthworkers, the service institutions, the health-insurance companies, the drug and hospital-supply companies, and government agencies. The needs of one or more of the provider groups and institutions include: job satisfaction and feelings of accomplishment, maintenance and improvement of income, profit, job security, prestige, power, efficiency, institutional perservation, and autonomy.

The Use of Needs Assessment in National-Health-Insurance Planning

This chapter will not analyze and rank by priority the various provider and patient needs outlined previously and propose an NHI design intended to meet the ranked needs. That is a complicated task that would take much more space than is presently available. What will be proposed is a basic NHI design that would make it possible for the program itself to carry out needs assessments on an ongoing basis, set priorities on the basis of those needs assessments, and, within the limits of available resources, make continual program adjustments to meet identified needs. The system would thus be able to directly incorporate planning information into program operations on a continuous basis, making it possible to achieve stated health and health-service goals. The current NHI proposals are based on some form of item-of-service reimbursement and the use of the regulatory approach to achieve desired goals. The assumption is made that none of the current NHI proposals would in fact be able to clearly and efficiently meet a set of stated goals, especially if those goals are concerned with improving health status and correcting deficiencies in medical-care organization.

A government-operated NHS system could of course directly and continually incorporate planning information into program operations. However, it is assumed that the NHS approach is not an acceptable one for the United States for the forseeable future for several reasons. First, it would appear that passage of an NHS act is politically impossible. Second, few if any government jurisdictions in this country have shown themselves capable of effectively operating medical-care services. There are good reasons for this: complex bureaucracies, non-health-related politically motivated legislative interference, civil-service rules, limitations on salaries related to nonhealthworker government salaries. Most important, however, is the third of several reasons why the NHS is not an acceptable alternative: the pauper stigma. The pauper stigma states that "poor is bad" and that poverty is the fault of the poor. Since the first government medical-care services in this country were for the poor, the pauper stigma was attached to them. It has remained attached, very firmly, in the public and the political mind over the years. Only revolutionary change can do away with the existence of the pauper stigma, one of the most basic tenets of capitalist ideology. This is not currently a feasible alternative.

The problem then is to come up with an approach that would allow for the direct application of planning information to health-services-system operation so that the focus on meeting identified needs could always be maintained without direct government operation. A further assumption is made here, that the numerous health providers are incapable of rational planning on their own and that government action in this area is necessary. Historical experience in this country speaks to the truth of this assumption. Furthermore, it is assumed that government will play an increasingly important role in the financing of health services, whether through taxes or the imposition and collection of uniform employer-employee contributions to pay for the cost of health services.

A classical approach to the achievement of stated goals and objectives is the contract mechanism. The buyer and seller of a product agree on product specifications and cost. Both are written down in a contract, which usually also contains means of enforcement of its terms. Herein proposed is the use of the contract mechanism as the basis of a national-health-insurance plan. A small-scale, partial prototype of such an approach existed in New York City during the 1970s. It was called "ghetto medicine." Before the contract mechanism for NHI is discussed, the major features of the New York City Ghetto Medicine program will be reviewed briefly.

The New York City Ghetto Medicine Program

Legislative History

In 1968 the New York state legislature created a program to permit local health departments to provide general medical services and charge for them [10].

The concept was based on one put forward by Herman Biggs when he was New York State Health Commissioner in 1920. The 1968 program was based on the assumption that the state's then-generous medicaid program would pay for the bulk of the ghetto-medicine program. A seemingly minor provision was written into the ghetto-medicine regulations, allowing local health departments to contract with voluntary agencies to provide general medical services in health-department facilities.

At the same time that the state legislature was passing ghetto medicine, however, it was sharply cutting back on medicaid funds. This greatly limited the development of the ghetto-medicine program as originally conceived. Only a few counties, including those comprising New York City, took part in it. By late 1969 the voluntary hospitals in New York City that had large outpatient departments were feeling the financial pinch of further medicaid-eligibility cuts and a state freeze on medicaid-reimbursement rates. They brought pressure on the governor, Nelson Rockefeller, to help them out. The governor did not want to call a special legislative session to deal with the problem. Using a great deal of imagination, it was determined that the ghetto-medicine legislation would do. Its regulations allowed health departments to contract for ambulatory services. The intent was to provide *new* services in health-department facilities, not pay for *existing* services in hospital facilities. Nevertheless, Governor Rockefeller found $6 million and gave it to the New York City Health Department under ghetto medicine to accomplish the latter goal.

The use of the original law in this way was probably illegal. It was never tested in court. The New York City program became moribound due to fund starvation in the late 1970s. While it was in operation, however, it taught some useful lessons.

Contracting for Quality

The New York City voluntary-hospital outpatient department support program was officially called the Ambulatory Care Program, ACP. Colloquially it continued to be referred to as "ghetto medicine." The original ghetto-medicine fiscal philosophy was to reimburse local health departments with state monies for 50 percent of the deficits incurred in the operation of direct medical-care programs. (Recall that it was originally assumed that medicaid would cover most of the costs so that the total deficits would be very small.) The 50-percent figure came from the historical 50 percent of cost that the state health department had paid to the local health department to support traditional local health-department services such as well-baby clinics and public-health nursing programs. Following this pattern, the city determined that it would pay the hospitals 50 percent of their outpatient-department deficits incurred after all third-party payments had been collected.

Following the provisions of the original ghetto-medicine regulations for support of operations by voluntary hospitals, the city health department invited all the city's voluntary hospitals that operated outpatient departments to apply for funds, which would be given to them under contract. A prototype contract was developed, and all participating hospitals were covered by it.

A major feature of both the contract negotiations and the contract-enforcement mechanism was the mandated existence of a community advisory board for each program. This resulted from a provision of the original state ghetto-medicine regulations which, contemplating a series of local health-department-operated ambulatory-care centers, required the existence of a consumer-majority advisory board for each program. In practice, a unique role was developed for the community boards, and their citywide representative body, which came to be known as the Ambulatory Care Consumer Advisory Committee. They were involved in negotiating the contract specifications and, with the health department, in enforcing the contracts through participation in the inspections that were regularly conducted by the health department. They were concerned with program outcomes, not the day-to-day details of program operations.

The roles were clearly delineated: The health department was the provider of funds, the principal determinant of program specifications, and the contract enforcer. The community boards participated in the establishment of program specifications and in the evaluation of hospital performance. The hospitals received the money, negotiated for recognition of their own needs in writing the contracts, and operated the programs. To make the community role significant, a health department that listened to and accepted advice was needed. That was the case. The contracts had the following major features:

Money was provided to maintain existing services, not establish new ones. However, there were required guarantees of maintenance of existing effort for funds received.

Global budgeting was established. Item-of-service reimbursement was discarded.

Required standards of service and care were set forth in some detail: "comprehensive, family orientation" was specified; there was to be a full-time director of ambulatory care; an individual-time appointment system was required; the hospital was required to provide to ghetto-medicine patients admitted from the outpatient service to the inpatient service the same level of care received by other admittees; a fee schedule had to be provided.

Regular health department inspections, which included provision for chart audits of a random sample of ambulatory patients, were provided for. The community board participated in these inspections.

Detailed "guidelines" for the structure and programs of the clinics and emergency departments were appended to the contracts and had the force of the contract. They dealt with such issues as basic required services, the time delay for new appointments, minimum time to be spent with patients, privacy, confidentiality, record systems, patient knowledge of condition and regimen, and patient education.

A guideline detailing the rights and responsibilities of the community board was also appended to the contract.

Toward the end of the program, specific weights were given to various elements of the contract program. Financial penalties, related to the weights, were exacted from the hospitals for noncompliance.

Inspections were undertaken on a regular basis. No comprehensive evaluation of the program was ever carried out. However, limited survey and anecdotal evaluations came up with generally positive results [10, pp. 90-97, 117-123]. There were noticeable improvemens in the quality of ambulatory services provided in those hospitals covered by the program. Furthermore, a useful and constructive role was developed for the community boards, with the active assistance of a health department interested in doing just that. An interesting sidelight on the program is that while the city pursued a very thorough and apparently effective inspection program for a service, which cost it no more than $10 million per year, it did little in the way of evaluating the use of its funds in another medical-care program that cost it many times that amount each year: medicaid.

In sum, the major features of the ghetto-medicine program were:

1. Government money was given to voluntary-agency providers of health services on a global-budgeting rather than an item-of-service basis.
2. Receipt of the money depended on agreement to a contract that contained quality-performance standards.
3. Community boards played a significant role in contract negotiations, performance evaluation, and contract enforcement.
4. The department of health provided the money, negotiated the contract, and enforced it.
5. The providers independently administered their own programs.

The contract mechanism as it existed in New York City's ghetto-medicine program holds promise as an alternative approach to NHI. It falls midway between all the current NHI proposals on the one hand, which rely on item-of-service reimbursement and regulations to achieve stated goals and objectives, and current NHS proposals, on the other hand, which rely on government ownership of the "means of production" and government operation of the system through some kind of community-board mechanism. In theory at least, the contract mechanism would allow the system to focus directly on meeting needs identified through planning techniques without entirely changing the patterns of ownership of the "means of production." At the same time it would provide a significant role for community representatives, in drawing up contract specifications and assessing outcomes, while allowing the providers to administer their own programs.

The Contract Mechanism for National Health Insurance

Basic Concepts

The basic concepts of the contract mechanism for NHI are very much like those of the New York City ghetto-medicine program. There is a set of problems that needs to be solved. The problems and desired means of solving them can be specified in contracts. It is useful to pay for health services through a global budget related to a program rather than on an item-of-service reimbursement basis. Contracts can be enforced jointly by government agencies and community representatives.

The outline of the system is fairly simple. Government would raise the funds necessary to pay for health services. It would then negotiate a series of contracts with providers as contractors, under which the contractors would agree to offer a set of services to the population for a given dollar amount. Much as group practice and independent practice association health-maintenance organizations do now, all providers would then market their services to consumers. All persons would be covered for a benefit package that would be determined nationally. Consumers would have free choice of contractor, but once having made their choice, as in present dual-choice situations, they would have to stay with the selected provider for a minimum period of time. Contract specifications would be determined using planning and quality-assessment data and mechanisms. Service priorities would be established. Advisory boards would be formed for each contractor consisting of patients serviced by that contractor. The boards would be party to contract negotiation and enforcement. There would be graded financial penalties for failure to meet contract specifications and rewards for excellent performance. Private ownership of the health-services sector would be maintained, but the people, through both the government and the advisory boards, would have a strong voice in deciding how their money is being spent.

Role of Government

This approach to NHI makes several assumptions about the role of government in it and in the health-care-delivery system in general. First, it assumes that the health and health-services problems briefly outlined in the first section of this chapter are worth solving, are soluble, and are serious enough to warrant government intervention to some degree. Health-services problems have changed little in this country since the publication of the *Final Report of the Committee on the Costs of Medical Care in 1932* [10], although the health problems have changed markedly. Voluntarism has had 50 years to deal with equal access to care, maldistribution of personnel and facilities, the importance of preventive services, fragmentation, and so on and so forth. The voluntary approach has not worked too well and has actually exacerbated certain problems such as cost containment and physician overspecialization. Second, this approach assumes that health-systems planning is an appropriate government function, along with standard setting and quality assurance. Third, it assumes that direct government operation of the health-care-delivery system is not a good idea, for the reasons outlined previously.

Federal Government. Under NHI by contract, government would have three principal roles: raiser of funds, negotiator of contracts, and enforcer of contracts. In theory, the entire job could be done by the federal government, either through the Department of Health and Human Services and its regional offices or through a newly established agency. This would be an enormous responsibility, however. The system would be very cumbersome and could easily become very inefficient. It would probably be better to give the federal government a role akin to what it does now in many health-related activities. It would raise and distribute funds to the primary contracting agencies, which would probably be at the state level. It would set national standards for contract specifications and establish upper and lower dollar limits within which contracts would be negotiated. It would determine the lump-sum dollar allocations to be made to each state (as it would under the Committee for National Health Insurance approach to NHI.) As in the HSA and PSRO systems, the federal government would act both as an arbiter of disputes and as the ultimate contract enforcer. Using information provided by the states, the HSAs, the PSROs, and other provider and consumer representatives, it would determine national health and health-services priorities from time to time. It would set the objectives for meeting identified needs and put those objectives into the national contract specifications. Thus the federal government would ensure the link between planning and implementation.

State Government. The primary contracting agencies could either be a set of new regional bodies, as in the Committee for National Health Insurance approach, or agencies based in the states. Since so much that is new would be required to implement this sytem in any case, it would probably be better to go with state agencies than to create yet another new agency, a regional health authority. The use of a state agency as the primary government arm in a national-health-insurance system is not new. It appears, for example, in the old American Hospital Association "Ameriplan," once upon a time introduced into Congress in 1975 by Congressman Al Ullman as "The National Health Care Services Reorganization and Financing Act: H.R. 1"[12]. (That proposal has since been withdrawn.) Under NHI by contract, the state agency could be the existing health department, the existing state health-planning-and-development agency, or a newly created state health commission à la the "Ameriplan." Whatever form it took, the state NHI agency would have to be freed from traditional state personnel practices and salary scales so that it could recruit personnel on the same bases that providers do. This measure would avoid the present situation in which state health-regulatory agencies recruit from a much smaller pool and pay their people much less than the institutions they are regulating.

The state health agency would have the primary responsibility for the determination of contract specifications within national guidelines, for negotiating contracts, for paying contractors, and for enforcing contract terms. In NHI by contract, the state health agencies would play the same role that the New York City Health Department did in ghetto medicine. However, while the primary *responsibility* would lie with the state health agencies, they might not do all the actual work themselves. In the larger states, local health departments could act as delegates, as in fact the New York Health Department did in the ghetto-medicine system. Furthermore, there are the existing private health-insurance companies to consider. At present, several hundred thousand people work in the health-insurance industry. No matter what other provisions were made, many of those people would be out of work in a system that no longer relied on item-of-service reimbursement and individual claims processing. However, it might be possible to create a new role for some insurance companies as delegates of state health agencies, participating in the contract system.

Funding Mechanism

The system would be supported by a combination of employer/employee contributions and general tax revenues. They would be collected by the federal government. Data on utilization, health and health services needs, the efficacy of diagnostic and therapeutic interventions, the quality of care, and costs would be gathered. Needs would be assessed, goals and objectives established, priorities set. The total national health budget would be capped by the funds collected. The total of the allocations to each state would obviously be fixed, but the level of allocation to each state would be subject to negotiation. Once the state agency received its allocation, it would have to negotiate contracts with all its providers for service to patients.

The negotiations that would take place under NHI by contract would obviously be extremely complex. Surely some of the people displaced from the insurance companies would find jobs in the NHI-negotiating system. The lead times on negotiations would have to be very long—longer than the customary government fiscal year. There would be the potential for whip-sawing the state health agency between the dollar limits and contract specifications set by the federal government and the demands of the institutional and individual providers. However, there would also be a strong motivation for providers to sign contracts: Everyone would be covered and would be paying for health services in one way or another. As in Great Britain, there would be few patients outside the system and to survive, most providers would have to be in it.

Contract Specifications

As has been pointed out several times previously, the most basic principle of this concept is that desired health-services outcomes should be (and can be) specified and that payment to providers should be linked to such specifications rather than merely to the fact that an item-of-service was given to a patient. The substantial role in contract specification, negotiation, and enforcement to be taken on by consumer representatives has also been covered. Obviously, a layering of boards at the several administrative levels would have to be worked out. In certain other plans that take a great deal of interest in consumer participation, a great deal of time is spent in discussing the details of the process of consumer participation. In this plan, establishing the principle of consumer involvement for the purpose of evaluating outcomes is most important. The details of the process can be developed later.

Data Collection and Input

NHI by contract would rely on the existing Health Systems Agnecies and Professional Standards Review Organizations in planning and quality assurance, respectively. The HSA approach is based on the principle of consumer-government-provider partnership. The PSRO approach is based on the principle of peer review backed up by government authority. Both principles are sound. The data collected by both systems is essential both for developing contract specifications and for contract enforcement. Health-status data would continue to be collected and analyzed by existing government agencies at the local, state, and national levels. They would advise the national health agency on health priorities and recommend health and disease-specific goals and objectives to be included in contract specifications. The evaluation of new and existing drugs, technologies, and procedures would be the responsibility of the Food and Drug Administration and the National Center for Health Care Technology.

They would advise the national health agency on the efficacy, safety, needs, and priorities for drugs, technologies, and procedures.

The Contractors

Most of the existing providers of service would be eligible to become either primary contractors or subcontractors. Presumably, the basic benefit package (not discussed in this chapter) would be built around primary-care outpatient services and secondary/tertiary-care specialist referral and inpatient services. If the primary contractor is principally in the inpatient-care business, it would have to either develop its own primary-care component or subcontract with a primary-care group or primary-care individual practitioners to provide such services. A quite similar concept is contained in the Health Care Corporation entity of Ameriplan, except that under Ameriplan, individuals were to have their own insurance policies, and providers were to be reimbursed on an item-of-service basis. If the primary contractor is principally in the outpatient business, it would subcontract for inpatient and specialty referral services as HMOs do now. All primary contractors would subcontract for drugs, testing, and those ancillary services that were covered. If long-term care were a covered benefit, primary contractors would subcontract for it as well.

Primary contractors would be paid on a global-budget basis. The global budget would be related to past and expected costs and service load. Maintenance of effort would be required. Increased enrollment would be rewarded, up to certain limits designed to encourage expansion and competition while discouraging patient exploitation, through the appropriate application of contract specifications. If the contract specifications for enrollment and services were met, and money were saved, the contractor would get to keep part of it for development purposes.

New services would receive start-up funds, after meeting certain requirements as is now the case under HMO legislation. New services would have enrollment and service-package goals and be given a specified time period in which to meet them. At the same time the contracting agency could decline to offer start-up funds for new services in adequately served areas, it could offer attractive contract incentives for new services established in underserved areas.

Private medical practice could be retained under NHI by contract, in several forms. Hospitals as primary contractors could subcontract with private physicians to offer ambulatory services in their own offices. This concept is to be found in Ameriplan. Independent practice associations could certainly compete as primary contractors, subcontracting for hospital services much as they and other HMOs do now. It would theoretically be possible for individual private practitioners to be primary contractors. However, they would have to subcontract for inpatient services, drugs, and so forth and would probably be overwhelmed by management problems. On the other hand, service corporations might be formed to provide the necessary subcontracted services to private physicians so that they could be primary contractors, as are general practitioners in Great Britain. The practice form would probably not turn out to be too much different from an IPA, however. Most specialists who now have referral practices would probably work directly for or subcontract to hospital or HMO primary contractors.

Certain health services would probably remain outside of the system, at least in the beginning. This group would consist of those federal services that take care of named population groups: The Veterans Administration hospitals; the Department of Defense health services; the Public Health Service medical-care services for Indians, Inuits, merchant seamen, and so forth; and the state services for named illnesses and conditions: mental disturbances and tuberculosis. Local government community hospitals would be absorbed into the system, however, eligible to be primary contractors. Special contracts would be written for university and other teaching hospitals, taking into account their special nature and the costs of their education and research functions. However, contract specifications would require that those functions be designed to be consistent with community needs for health services.

Contract Enforcement

The pattern of contract enforcement would follow the ghetto-medicine example. The state health agency and its local delegates would be charged with this responsibility. The community health board attached to each primary contractor would play a major role in the process. PSRO, HSA, FDA, and National Center for Health Care Technology data, recommendations and decisions would be very important in the decision-making process, along with the results of direct inspections.

Advantages of National Health Insurance by Contract

NHI by contract is based on the concept that the planning principle of beginning program design with needs assessment is most productive in terms of improving the health of the people, which is assumed to be the most important goal of the health-care-delivery system. It provides the opportunity to plan programs by establishing goals and objectives and also provides the means for directly achieving them, without complete government ownership and operation of the system. It provides the opportunity to deal directly with the three principal problems presently facing the U.S. health-care-delivery system: cost control, quality improvement, and implementing a comprehensive health-promotion and disease-prevention program.

NHI by contract enables the direct focusing of effort and expenditure. A fair degree of fine tuning can be accomplished. It leaves behind the present reliance on regulation and prayer to achieve program goals and objectives. There is a clear role for community advisory boards, focusing on outcomes, not process. It creates a clear role for state and local health departments, in addition to their traditional one of providing community health services. It does away with item-of-service reimbursement, which is such a stimulus to overutilization and provider abuse.

NHI by contract does not begin with benefit packages and decisions on copayment, which so many other approaches to NHI do. It begins with the establishment of planning principles and assumes that benefit packages will be developed and decisions on copayment made *after* needs are assessed, goals and objectives are set, and the amount of available funds is determined.

NHI by contract is consistent with the "American way." The independence of the providers is maintained. This provider independence is balanced by public direction of the expenditure of public funds. It is in fact somewhat similar to the Health Care Corporation/State Health Commission of the old Ameriplan, with the substitution of global budgeting for item-of-service reimbursement. Finally, it provides for serious competition among providers, an element being called for now by many prominent health economists. The competition, however, would be around who is doing the best job of achieving stated goals and objectives, not who is offering the cheapest product.

Disadvantages of National Health Insurance by Contract

The system would probably be quite cumbersome, especially for the first few years. Negotiations would be extremely complex and long lead times, to which few Americans are accustomed, would be required for their conclusion. The providers would be called on to make major functional and psychological changes, although not of the same magnitude as would be required under the national-health-service approach. Behavioral change would be required among patients as well, although recent experience with the burgeoning HMO indicates that patient-behavior change would come more easily than provider-behavior change. And after all, from the perspective of most patients, NHI by contract would look much like a vastly expanded HMO system. There would be a large redundant staff in the health-insurance industry as individual-claims processing became a thing of the past. However, there would be many positions in negotiating bodies at many levels and in inspectorates.

When Will National Health Insurance Come?

It is currently popular in some circles to say that NHI is "an idea whose time has gone." In the stock market, the bull market usually begins just as the "little guy" turns bearish, and vice versa. That could well happen in the history of NHI too. When we have stopped looking for it, it will appear. It is popular in some circles to say that NHI is too expensive, that the nation "cannot afford" to have it. The truth is just the opposite. With the skyrocketing costs, questionable quality, and massive misallocation of resources that occur under the present voluntary, "free" system, the nation annot afford *not* to have it. However, getting it is not that simple. The provider control groups are very powerful, and in an era of legislation by special interest, they have a great deal of influence.

The two most powerful control groups in the health-care-delivery system are the physicians and the hospitals. Major changes in the system have taken place in the past when the physicians and/or the hospitals wanted or needed those changes, for example, the reinstitution of medical licensing laws in the late nineteenth century and the development of voluntary hospital insurance during the Great Depression. NHI will come when one or the other or both of those groups want it or need it. The hospitals will want it as an increasing number of them go bankrupt, as happened in Great Britain just before the institution of the National Health Service. The physicians will want it when their number is so large that they will no longer be able to sell all the product they can collectively produce, as they can now. With a majority of them being private entrepreneurs, the competition would be chaotic. The shelter of a secure, if somewhat smaller income would be sought. We are likely to encounter this situation by the middle of the 1990s.

Thus the United States will probably have NHI by the year 2000, with so-called catastrophic health insurance and the expansion of welfare health insurance as an interim step. NHI by contract as an alternative to present proposals, in an effort to design a system that focuses not on processes but on outcomes.

Notes

1. *Healthy People: The Surgeon General's Report on Health Promotion and Disease Prevention: 1979.* Washington, D.C.: USDHEW (PHS) Pub. No. 79-55071.

2. I have reviewed with references the current problems of the U.S. health-care-delivery system in chap. 3 of my book *Medical Mystery: The Training of Doctors in the United States* (New York: Norton, 1979).

3. J.W. Farquhar, *The American Way of Life Need Not Be Hazardous to Your Health* (New York: Norton, 1978).

4. R.L. Kane; Josephine M. Kasteler; and Robert M. Gray, *The Health Gap: Medical Services and the Poor* (New York: Springer, 1976); USDHEW, *Health of the Disadvantaged: Chart Book.* (Hyattsville, Md., DHEW Pub. No. (HRA) 77-628, 1977).

5. R.M. Gibson, "National Health Expenditures, 1978," *Health Care Financing Review,* Summer, 1979, table 1.

6. A. Donabedian, "The Quality of Medical Care," chap. 6 in *Health, United States: 1978* (Washington, D.C.: USDHEW, Pub. No. (PHS) 78-1232, 1978).

7. R. Roemer, et al. *Planning Urban Health Services: From Jungle to System* (New York: Springer, 1975).

8. J. Lebow, "Consumer Assessments of the Quality of Care," *Medical Care* 12 (1974):328; G.L. Engle, "The Care of the Patient: Art of Science?" *The Johns Hopkins Medical Journal* 140 (1977):222-232.

9. L.W. Green, "How to Evaluate Health Promotion," *Hospitals* (October 1979):106; D.M. Vickery, "Is It a Change for the Better?" *Hospitals* (October 1979):87; C.I. Cohen and E.J. Cohen "Health Education: Panacea, Pernicious or Pointless?" *New England Journal of Medicine* 299 (1978):718.

10. I have described ghetto medicine in detail in chap. 5 to 7 of *Quality-control of Ambulatory Care: A Task for Health Departments* (New York: Springer, 1977).

11. The Committee on the Costs of Medical Care, *Medical Care for the American People* (Chicago: University of Chicago Press, 1932). Reprinted Washington, D.C.: USDHEW, 1970.

12. Al Ullman, "The National Health Care Services Reorganization and Financing Act–H.R. 1," *Congressional Record,* 14 January 1975.

9 National Health Insurance and Beyond

Joseph C. Morreale

One of the foremost public-policy debates in the 1970s in the United States focused on the possible adoption of a national-health-insurance system. This debate had many causes including rapidly escalating health-care costs, the recognition of the inequitable distribution of health-care resources, the greater public role in health-care programs put forth during the 1960s, and a sense of health care being a basic public right. Various proposals have been made by all of the vested interest groups, but as yet no one program has gained sufficient support. And so, the United States continues to spend increasing amounts on health care reaching almost $200 billion during the twelve months ending March 1979 and amounting to 9 percent of the GNP.[1]

In the meantime most western industrialized, developed countries have already adopted some form of national health insurance. Canada is one of the most recent of these nations, having implemented and experimented with a national insurance system for about ten years. Since in many ways Canada is very similar to the United States in terms of its history, culture, and economic, social, and political institutions, the Canadian experience with national health insurance offers some interesting insights into its potential impact in the United States. The U.S. experience with medicare and medicaid can point to some further insights. Of particular concern in this chapter will be consideration of cost, access, and equity issues. In addition, some more fundamental political-economic issues related to health and health care in the United States will be raised and analyzed in terms of consideration of public-health policy. And finally, a new health policy relating to these more fundamental issues will be offered.

The Canadian Experience with National Health Insurance

The Canadians developed a national-health-insurance system in stages between 1958 and 1968. In 1958 the federal government passed the Hospital Insurance and Diagnostic Services Act, which provided comprehensive and uniform coverage for hospital and diagnostic services through joint federal-provincial funding. In 1966 the federal government enacted the Canadian Assistance Plan, which added medical and surgical insurance coverage for people on public assistance. And finally, in 1968 it extended this coverage to the general population through the Medical Care Act. By 1971 all provinces had adopted this plan so that virtually all the Canadian population was covered by a federal-provincial shared financial system of comprehensive health care covering hospital, diagnostic, medical, and surgical services. Since then, dental and eye care have been introduced in many of the provinces. We will focus on three important effects: health-care costs, access to health care, and financial equity.

Cost

Trends in the cost of health and medical care related to the passage of Canadian national health insurance have begun to be detected. Professor Robert Evans has shown that the pattern of increase in health-care expenditures directly relates to extensions in health-insurance coverage in Canada.[2] He finds that the largest increase in hospital-care spending as a proportion of personal income occurred between 1960 and 1965, and medical-care spending increased its proportion during the period 1965-1970 with acceleration in this trend in 1971. Each respective period corresponds to the adoption of the hospital-insurance plan and the national-health-insurance program by the provinces.

This author has studied changes in health-care expenditures in Canada as a whole and in detail in Quebec in the pre- and post-national-health-insurance periods.[3] (See table 9-1.) The results indicate that after the introduction of national health insurance, an initial sharp increase occurred in health-care expenditures caused mainly by increased expenditures on physicians services. This increase shows that more resources (as measured by health-care expenditures per capita, as a percent of GNP, and as a percent of personal income) were devoted to health care. There followed a period of slowdown in the rate of increase of expenditures (1971-1973), but afterward there has been further acceleration of this rate. In general, if a comparison is made of the five-year period during which passage of medicare occurred with the prior five-year period for each province, it appears that for most of the provinces the percentage increase in health expenditures is significant. Moreover, an accelerating trend in the percentage change in health expenditures is seen in the five-year postmedicare period in most of the provinces.

Access

The few published studies for certain provinces in Canada that have analyzed access to health care after the introduction of national health insurance indicate that some redistribution of medical-care services toward the lower income groups occurred. Badgley et al. did a pre- and postanalysis of the utilization of health care of people in a small town in Saskatchewan for the years 1960 and 1965.[4] The found that physician utilization as measured by family contact with a physician increased and that people with low income and little education saw their physicians more readily for health care. They also found that those with higher incomes and more education used specialists more frequently. Beck also studied the Saskatchewan experience but for the years 1965 and 1968.[5] He attempted to identify the percentage of the population by income class that did not contact a physician in a given year. His results show that the greatest decrease occurred for the lowest income groups, and so he concludes that medical care became more equitably distributed. However, he also points out that this reduced disparity is primarily for general practitioners but that access to specialists increased for all income groups with the higher income groups still having much greater access to medical specialist's services.

Enterline et al. studied changes in the distribution of access to physician services across income classes in Montreal pre- and postmedicare (1969-1970 and 1971-1972).[6] In their analysis of physician visits per person for five income classes, they found that there was a significant redistribution of physician visits toward the lower income groups. Moreover, they analyzed the changes in these different groups seeking medical care based on a set of medical symptoms. Prior to medicare a smaller percent of the lowest three income classes having those symptoms would see a physician than the highest two classes. After medicare this relationship disappeared so that the lower three income groups saw physicians at least as frequently for the same set of symptoms as the upper two income classes.

Equity

To this author's knowledge, the only study of the impact on financial equity of the introduction of national health insurance is his own in Quebec.[7] This study focused on the distributional impact of Quebec medicare on medical-care costs pre- and post-national health insurance (1969-1970 and 1971-1972). In the premedicare period estimates were made of the financing of medical and surgical services through premiums paid to private health insurers, out-of-pocket payments for deductibles, coinsurance factors, and uncovered services, and the incidence of federal-provincial shared revenues across income classes. In the postmedicare period, estimates were made of the incidence of provincial payroll tax and federal-provincial shared revenues across income classes. Also real (waiting time) costs of obtaining medical care for both periods were estimated across income classes. The results of this study showed that medical-care costs for most income groups (excluding the lowest one) increased sharply and the proportion of family income spent on medical care rose significantly. However, medical-care costs display a sharper increase for higher income groups than lower ones. Moreover, it was found that the range of average medical-care costs across income classes widened, and the incidence of medical-care costs for various income classes became much more progressive. Therefore, there was evidence that medical-care costs had become more equitably distributed.

The U.S. Experience with Public Health-Insurance Programs

The previous section analyzed the impact of publicly financed national health insurance in Quebec and Canada on health-care costs, financial equity, and access. We now turn to an analysis of the impact of public health-care financing in the United States. To date, U.S. health-care-financing policy has primarily focused on the indigent population. Since 1966 the poor have been covered by a jointly (federal-state) administered and financed program (medicaid) and the elderly have been covered by a federally administered and financed health-insurance program for the aged (medicare). The cost of these two programs in fiscal year 1978 reached $43.3 billion amounting to over one quarter of all spending on health in the United States.[8]

Cost

Table 9-1 displays data on total health expenditures, public health expenditures, and private health expenditures in the United States for the period 1960-1975. A comparison of the percentage changes in this increase of health-care expenditures between 1960-1965 and 1965-1970 shows that the rate was 50 percent higher in the postmedicare and medicaid period than in the premedicare and medicaid period. Moreover, individual annual data demonstrate that the acceleration in health-care expenditures began suddenly in fiscal year 1967. It can be seen that the higher rate of increase persists for the period 1970-1975. In a recent related study, Anderson et al. also analyzed the rate of increase of medical-care expenditures in the United States pre- and postmedicare and medicaid.[9] The main finding from this study is that the overall rate of increase was twice as high in the postmedicare-medicaid period relative to the premedicare-medicaid period.

Access

Since the passage of medicare and medicaid, there has been a significant increase in utilization of health-care services by the poor and the elderly. Davis reports that in 1964, physician visits per person per year for high-income families were 20 percent higher than for poor families, but in 1974, low-income families were 13 percent greater.[10] Also the gap in physician utilization by poor children versus those in the higher income families was significantly reduced. Major

Table 9-1
Total Health Expenditures and Percent Changes in Health Expenditures: Quebec, Canada, and the United States (1960-1975)
(expenditures in millions of dollars)

	1960	1965	1970	1971	1972	1973	1974	1975	1960-1965	1965-1970	1970-1975
Quebec											
Health expenditures	528	914	1581	1839	1983	2246	2647	2956	—	—	—
Percent changes in health expenditures[a]	—	—	—	16.3	7.8	13.3	17.9	11.7	73.0	73.0	87.0
Canada											
Health expenditures	2155	3362	6081	6949	7566	8456	9912	11,749	—	—	—
Percent changes in health expenditures[a]	—	—	—	14.3	8.9	11.8	17.2	18.5	78.5	80.9	93.2
United States											
Health expenditures	25,856	38,892	69,201	77,162	86,687	95,383	106,321	123,716	—	—	—
Percent changes in health expenditures[a]	—	—	—	11.5	12.3	10.0	11.5	16.4	50.4	77.9	78.7
Percent changes in public health expenditures[a]	—	—	—	13.3	16.3	9.5	13.2	26.2	49.1	166.3	106.2
Percent changes in private health expenditures[a]	—	—	—	10.4	10.0	10.3	10.4	10.1	50.9	49.2	62.9

Sources: Department of National Health and Welfare, Health Expenditure and Resources Division, Unpublished tables, Ottawa, Canada, table IV. U.S. Department of Health, Education, and Welfare, Health Care Financing Administration, "HCFA Health Notes," Washington, D.C., May 1978, table 1.
[a] Author's estimates.

gains were also made by the poor in the percent seeing a physician in the previous two years and in the percent of women receiving prenatal physician care.

Yet despite these gains, persistent inequities still remain.[11] There are still problems of access for many poor and elderly. Medicaid does not provide medical services for all poor persons but only for those falling within specified welfare categories. Moreover, many are still excluded from coverage with poor blacks and people living in the South being disproportionately represented among the excluded. In addition, the poor are not receiving the same kind of medical care as middle- and upper-class Americans. The poor are much more likely to receive care from general practitioners and from outpatient departments, and the poor have to wait much longer priods of time and travel longer distances to receive care. Racial discrimination still interferes with equal benefits under medicare and medicaid. Payments per white recipient are substantially higher than payments for black recipients. And finally, though there is greater equality in utilization of medical services among income classes, this may still not represent the achievement of equal access. Poor people generally have more severe health problems than higher income people, and people receiving welfare are less healthy as a whole than other people. Moreover, Davis and Reynolds report that when adjustment is made for health status for the elderly, physician visits and hospital care increase uniformly with income.[12]

Equity

Even if medicare and medicaid have assisted poor and elderly people as a whole in receiving medical care, there is still an uneven distribution of financial burden and benefits among eligible people.[13] In 1970 people with incomes below $3500 paid virtually the same fraction of their income on medical care as in 1963. Moreover, people with incomes below $2000 spent almost 15 percent of their income on medical services in 1970 compared to only 4.4 percent for all people. Benefits from the physician's portion of medicare are particularly unequally distributed among income classes. Elderly with family income above $15,000 per year receive twice as much under Medicare Part B as those with incomes below $5000. Moreover, the deductible and coinsurance provisions of the physician portion of medicare constitute significant deterrents to the use of medical-care services by the elderly poor. And finally, Anderson et al. reported the effects of price increases across income classes in the pre- and post-medicare-medicaid periods.[14] Breaking the population into low-, middle-, and high-income classes, they found that prior to medicare and medicaid, the medical-care price increases were proportional across income classes. However, after the introduction of medicare and medicaid, these price increases were regressive.

Lessons Concerning the National-Health-Insurance Strategy

From the preliminary results seen in studies of the Canadian national-health-insurance system and of the U.S. medicare and medicaid programs, some important lessons can be learned concerning future adoption of publicly financed health insurance in the United States. First, the adoption of publicly financed health insurance in the United States would probably bring forth a sudden initial increase in health-care expenditures. Not only did this occur in Canada after the passage of the Canadian Medical Care Act but was also evident in the United States after the adoption of medicare and medicaid. Second, although this rapid initial increase in health-care expenditures would not be maintained, a higher rate of increase in health-care expenditures would be seen, Based on recently published estimates through 1975, this outcome is evident in Canada as a whole and across the provinces. Moreover, the U.S. experience with medicare and medicaid has displayed an acceleration in health-care expenditures, although this probably reflects the specific, high-need populations covered by the U.S. programs. Third, access to health care would be more equitably distributed. Based on the comparative studies of accessibility in Canada before and after national health insurance and the growing number of studies in the United States on medicare and medicaid, the poor and lower income classes would probably gain some more accessibility to health care than they have at present. And finally, there would be some redistribution of the financial burden of health care across income classes. The experiences in Quebec with medicare and in the United States with medicare and medicaid seem to indicate that health-care expenses should be less burdensome on lower income groups.

We must also recognize the important limitations of the national-health-insurance strategy. First, it will not solve the health-care cost-escalation problem. Much has been made about the relative rates of growth of health-care expenditures versus GNP in Canada and the U.S. Table 9-2 shows that though Canada and the United States both spent about 6 percent of their respective GNPs on health expenditures in 1965, ten years later Canada's percentage (7.2) is substantially below the U.S. percentage (8.5). This might be interpreted as more cost control in Canada under national health insurance. However, more careful analysis shows that (1) the rate of increase of Canadian health expenditures has been much higher than that of the United States, and (2) the more rapid rate of growth of the Canadian economy vis-à-vis the U.S. economy has diluted the impact of relatively higher health-care expenditure increases.

Second, national health insurance will not correct the maldistribution of health-care resources sufficiently to guarantee access to health care for all. It will modify the present inequities but many problems will remain. We have seen that unequal access still exists in Canada under national health insurance and also in the United States with its special public programs for the elderly and poor. The fundamental problem is that national health insurance is a

Table 9-2
Health Expenditures and Gross National Product: Quebec, Canada, and the United States (1965-1975)
(billions of dollars)

	1965	1970	1971	1972	1973	1974	1975	1970-1975 (Geometric) (Mean)
Quebec								
Gross provincial product	—	21.1	22.8	26.3	29.9	35.2	39.6	—
Health expenditures as a percent of GPP	—	7.5	8.1	7.5	7.5	7.5	7.5	—
Percent change in GPP[a]	—	—	8.0	15.0	13.6	17.7	12.3	12.9
Percent change in health expenditures[a]	—	—	16.3	7.8	13.3	17.9	11.7	12.9
Canada								
Gross national product	53.4	85.7	93.3	106.2	124.4	147.0	163.8	—
Health expenditures as a percent of GNP	6.0	7.1	7.4	7.1	6.8	6.7	7.2	—
Percent change in GNP[a]	—	—	8.9	13.8	17.1	18.1	11.4	13.4
Percent change in health expenditures[a]	—	—	14.3	8.9	11.8	17.2	18.5	13.7
United States								
Gross national product	658.0	960.2	1019.8	1111.8	1238.6	1361.2	1454.5	—
Health expenditures as a percent of GNP	5.9	7.2	7.6	7.8	7.7	7.8	8.5	—
Percent change in GNP[a]	—	—	6.2	9.0	11.4	9.8	6.8	12.1
Percent change in health expenditures[a]	—	—	11.5	12.3	10.0	11.5	16.4	12.1

Sources: Department of Industry and Commerce, *The Economic Situation of Quebec*, Quebec City, Quebec, 1976, tables 3 and 6, pp. 13 and 15 (for 1972-1975), and Ibid., 1974, tables 3 and 6, pp. 13 and 16 (for 1970-1971); Department of National Health and Welfare, *National Health Expenditures in Canada 1960-1973*, Ottawa, Canada, April 1975, table 52, p. 62; Department of National Health and Welfare, Ibid.; U.S. Department of HEW, Ibid.

[a] Author's estimates.

demand-side strategy. Of particular concern is the problem of who should set the priorities in the health-care system. Presently health professionals establish these priorities, but given the persistence of inequities in their priorities, increased public and/or consumer control is needed. Third, national health insurance only somewhat alters the regressive and inequitable method of paying for health care. From the experience in Canada and the proposals put forth in the United States, emphasis is placed on financing national health insurance with regressive taxes (like the employer-employee payroll tax). Also though Canada has rejected the use of deductibles and coinsurance factors, most U.S. proposals have incorporated such utilization deterrents in their plans, thereby compounding the regressivity of the national-health-insurance strategy.

In addition to these limitations, a few notes of caution are being expressed in Canada about national health insurance. Increasingly more emphasis is being placed on the supply side of the market. In analyzing the rising cost of health care, Evans has concluded,

> What we observe, and what generates expense, is not demand in the economist's sense but utilization. . .[which]. . . is the outcome of patient demand and physician behavior. . . . The role of national health insurance may simply have been to relax further any market constraints on how physicians manipulate utilization to generate income.[15]

In fact, Enterline et al. studied the impact of Quebec medicare on physician behavior and discovered that physicians reduced their working hours, and there was an overall decline in patient contacts.[16] However, contacts with patients in the office sharply increased while a sharp decline in home visits and telephone consultations was seen. Moreover, Evans, this author, and others have observed a sharp increase in physician incomes across all provinces after the adoption of medicare.[17] As Evans has argued, "insurance changes only the demand side of health care—the supply side is crucial. The hardest part of the job lies ahead."[18]

And finally, many have begun to question the further pay off in improved health status from increased expenditures on health care. For example, in looking at health-care expenditures versus mortality rates, Leveson finds that there has been a rapid decline in mortality rates from the late 1930s to the early 1950s but that the rate of health improvement slowed thereafter. Yet, the rate of growth of health expenditures accelerated from the 1950s to the present.[19] There was substantial evidence that health spending has a much larger effect on the mortality of infants and children than on the general population. And in the period since 1973, a renewed decline in mortality occurred at the same time that there was a slowdown in health-care expenditures. The McKinlays analyzed the decline in mortality in the United States between 1900-1973.[20] Like Leveson, they also find little relationship between accelerating health-care expenditures and declines in mortality rates and generally conclude that medical measures have contributed little to the overall decline in mortality in the United States over this century. Moreover, they show that the beginning of the sharp rise in medical-care expenditures began after nearly all (92 percent) of the modern decline in mortality during this century had already occurred. Another recent study by Newhouse and Friedlander found that variations in the amount of health resources available across 39 metropolitan areas of the United States had no systematic effect on any of six indicators of ill health.[21] And finally, after reviewing the recent health-economics literature, Fuchs has concluded, "when the state of medical science and other health determining variables are held constant, the marginal contribution of medical care to health is very small in modern nations."[22]

Simultaneously with the increasing questioning of the relationship of health care to improving health status has been an increase in research concerning various social, economic, political, and environmental determinants of health status. Attention has focused on four key factors that have significant effects on health status: economic inequality, class structure, education, and environmental pollution.

The U.S. capitalist economy results in inequality in income and wealth, and this income and wealth distribution has remained constant over the past 30 years.[23] Since, in general, resources flow to those areas with the greatest ability to pay, such economic inequality contributes to an unequal distribution of health-care resources. Moreover, there is a demonstrable inverse relationship between socioeconomic level and health status.[24]

This income and wealth inequality leads to a class structure in the economy that is reflected in the health-care system. Analysis of the boards of trustees of foundations, medical teaching institutions, and community hospitals shows that there is a predominance of the representatives of financial and corporate capital.[25] In addition, the existence of class structure is mirrored in differences in the health status of the various classes. The working class shows greater incidence of mortality and morbidity and suffers from proportionally more chronic conditions than the upper class.[26]

Much has been made of the positive correlation between educational level and good health, and some have suggested an increased emphasis on raising educational levels to bring about improved health status.[27] Yet inequities in education are also reflections of the general economic inequality. Economic inequality results in unequal access to high-quality educational institutions and also leads to unequal educational achievement.[28]

And finally, there is increasing awareness of the interrelationship of the economic system, environmental pollution, and human health. Capitalism requires material economic growth for its survival, and yet such needs generate increased levels of pollution which are harmful to the population. Urban air-pollution levels have been linked to heightened incidences of a variety of respiratory diseases and are related to problems of heart attacks, cancers of of the stomach and lungs.[29] The unequal distribution of income, wealth, and power is also mirrored in the unequal incidence of social costs of pollution.[30] Economic necessity forces many of the poor and near-poor to live in harmful environments while many of the rich are environmentally better off. Blue-collar workers likewise suffer more than professional workers because they are more likely to work in and live near polluting plants and factories.

Conclusion: A New Health-Policy Strategy

The results of the previous analysis has lead this author to the conclusion that publicly financed national health insurance is only a small step toward achieving such goals as control of increases in health-care expenditures, access to health care for all, equitable financial incidence of health-care costs, and improved health factors. A much broader view of factors that influence health status and a more fundamental change in our health-care system is needed. We must recognize the overriding importance of environmental factors in regard to health, such as life style, ecological deterioration, education, and nutrition. There is growing evidence of the overall and distributional effects of these factors on health status. Moreover, we must realize the need for a supply strategy to correct the maldistribution of health-care resources that the present system has brought about. And finally, we should take heed of the new concerns of Canadian officials and the needed changes that they recognize from their experience with national health insurance.

In light of these remarks, I would like to propose a more comprehensive and more fundamental change in the health-care system of the United States: A national health program of community health, education, and care centers. This community organization concept would combine the traditional functions of the public health department, neighborhood health center, hospital outpatient department, and private medical clinics. The center would have five functions:

1. To monitor and make the community aware of key environmental, occupational, social, and economic factors that affect the local community's health status
2. To educate the local community on those factors that increase their risk to disease and promote their given health status
3. To do research on local health problems and publish their results in a periodic newsletter for their population
4. To provide basic primary medical care and public health activities to improve and protect the health status of their population
5. To take an advocacy role on behalf of the community with regard to recognized health hazards in their community

Each center would be organized on the county level and be responsible for a community of between 10,000 and 25,000 people. In rural areas with less than this size population, multicounty cooperation would be required. In major urban areas, these centers would be in specific neighborhoods and/or recognized sections of the city. The people would retain the right to select whatever center they felt provided the best services. However, in most cases these centers would probably become regional monopolies, and therefore there is a need for them to be publicly controlled and nonprofit.

The initial funds for these centers could be provided through government and/or private charitable start-up grants. The centers' operating funds would be obtained by a national health tax on all firms producing a health hazard to workers or communities and redistributed across these centers to achieve equal real per-capita expenditure on health status. As firms cleaned up their environmental, occupational, and other health hazards, the population would be under less health hazard, and the centers would require less funds. Such a tax would also provide an incentive to the local center to uncover health hazards. Since the centers would be publicly funded, their services would be "free" to the users. The public would still retain the right to see private fee-for-service physicians and other health professionals, but such services would be paid for out of pocket.

This author feels that such a program of community health, education, and care centers would go a long way toward creating a much more equitable distribution of health-care services and health-care financing and also would help to reduce health risks and health-care expenditures.

However, to fully achieve greater equity in the maintenance of health status and efficiency in the allocation of scarce resources devoted to health maintenance would require more fundamental structural changes in our society. We must begin to emphasize quality of life and material sufficiency.[31] At present, advanced industrialized countries are enamored with quantity of production and economic growth as *the* determinants of human happiness. Such a view emphasizes people's insatiable wants and results in increasing destruction of the life-supporting environment and "materialist alienation" of the population. In my view, these characteristics are antihealth. Material sufficiency means obtaining the maximum well-being with minimum consumption and a stress on "quality of being."

Tied to this first change is the need to adopt a more humane, environmentally preserving technology. We have accepted the idea that increasing use of energy and natural resources is directly related to increasing affluence and improved well-being. Yet, the resulting increase in air, water, and land pollution clearly leads to reduced health status of our population. What is needed is a turning to alternative technologies stressing renewable and less polluting resources. Also stress on more labor-intensive as opposed to capital-intensive production processes would foster this effort and simultaneously stimulate employment of the population.

A third change is the need for increased emphasis on the independence of the individual and the cooperativeness of the community. We have brought forth a society that makes people dependent on professionals for very basic services that they could, and at one time did, provide for themselves. Yet simultaneously, we have also destroyed the sense of community needed when individuals do have to work together. In my view, the community, health, education, and care center is an example of such an effort. In addition, a more general decentralized control of industry is required. To help foster the goals of community and self-reliance, decision-making power would have to be placed much more in the hands of the people. This could be accomplished by instituting a limit on corporate size or encouraging community ownership of economic enterprises. In either case more people would be directly involved in setting the priorities of the economic institutions.

Intertwined with these changes is a requirement for a much more equal distribution of income and wealth and reduction in social-class differences. The evidence concerning the effect of inequality in income and wealth and the maintenance of social classes on the health of different groups is clear. Hence, some maximum and minimum limit of income and wealth should be established through the taxing system. Since there would be no incentive to go beyond the maximum limit, greater opportunities for economic pursuit would exist for the not-so-wealthy and therefore for a much greater proportion of the population. Since a family could not fall below the minimum lower limit, much greater economic security would be provided and a higher level of health status would be guaranteed.

In conclusion, national health insurance will only achieve modest success in our desire to guarantee access to services, equity in financial burden, and improved efficiency—if it achieves these effects at all. If we are serious about these goals, then we will need to consider a program that brings about changes in our health-care-delivery system. However, more important, these goals will require much more fundamental changes in our society. Either we make these fundamental changes now, or we try other more limited means only to find that these changes are still required. The choice is ours.

Notes

1. Health Care Financing Administration, *Health Care Financing Trends* 1(No. 1) (Fall 1979):1.

2. Robert Evans, "Beyond the Medical Market Place: Expenditure, Utilization, and Pricing of Insured Health Care in Canada," in Richard Rosett, ed., *The Role of Health Insurance in the Health Services Sector* (New York: National Bureau of Economic Research, 1976), pp. 448-449.

3. Joseph C. Morreale, "The Cost of National Health Insurance: The Province of Quebec," *Inquiry* 14 (December 1977):330-340; Joseph C.

Morreale, "The Distributional Effects of National Health Insurance in Quebec," *Journal of Health Politics, Policy and Law* 1 (Winter 1978):479-507; and Joseph C. Morreale, "The Quebec Experience, The Canadian Context, and Lessons for the U.S.," *Inquiry* 15 (September 1978):291-298.

4. Robin F. Badgley et al, "The Impact of Medicare in Wheatville, Saskatchewan, 1960-1965," *Canadian Journal of Public Health* 58 (March 1967).

5. R.G. Beck, "Economic Class and Access to Physician Services under Public Medical Care Insurance," *International Journal of Health Services* 1 (No. 3) (1973).

6. Philip E. Enterline et al. "The Distribution of Medical Services Before and After 'Free' Medical Care: The Quebec Experience," *New England Journal of Medicine* 289 (29 November 1973):1174-1178.

7. Joseph C. Morreale, "The Distributional Effects of National Health Insurance in Quebec."

8. Robert Gibson, "National Health Expenditures, 1978," *Health Financing Review* 1 (Summer 1979):1.

9. Ronald Andersen et al. "Rates and Correlates of Expenditure Increases for Personal Health Services: Pre- and Post-Medicare and Medicaid," *Inquiry* 13 (June 1976):136-144.

10. Karen Davis, "Medicaid Payments and Utilization of Medical Services by the Poor," *Inquiry* 13 (June 1976):126.

11. For a more thorough discussion of these inequities see Karen Davis, "Medicaid Payments," pp. 122-135; Karen Davis, *National Health Insurance: Benefits, Costs and Consequences* (Washington D.C.: The Brookings Institution, 1975), pp. 41-55; and Karen Davis and Roger Reynolds, "The Impact of Medicare and Medicaid on Access to Medical Care," in Richard Rosett, ed., *The Role of Health Insurance in the Health Service Sector* (New York: National Bureau of Economic Research, 1976):391-425.

12. Karen Davis and Roger Reynolds, "The Impact of Medicare and Medicaid," pp. 411-416.

13. Karen Davis, "Medical Payments and Utilization of Medical Services by the Poor," pp. 133-134; and Karen Davis, *National Health Insurance: Benefits, Costs, and Consequences*, pp. 51-52.

14. Ronald Andersen et al. "Rates and Correlates of Expenditure Increases for Personal Health Services: Pre- and Post-Medicare and Medicaid," pp. 142-43.

15. Robert Evans, "Beyond the Medical Marketplace: Expenditure, Utilization, and Pricing of Insured Health Care in Canada," in Robert Rosett, ed., *The Role of Health Insurance,* p. 476.

16. Philip E. Enterline, "Effects of 'Free' Medical Care on Medical Practice: The Quebec Experience," *New England Journal of Medicine* 288 (31 May 1973):1152-1155.

17. Robert Evans, "Beyond the Medical Marketplace: Expenditure,

Utilization, and Pricing of Insured Health Care in Canada," in Richard Rosett, ed., *The Role of Health Insurance*, pp. 468-472.

18. Ibid., p. 480.

19. Irving Leveson, "Some Policy Implications of the Relationship Between Health Services and Health," *Inquiry* 16 (Spring 1979):9-21.

20. John B. McKinlay and Sonja McKinlay, "The Questionable Contribution of Medical Measures to the Decline of Mortality in the United States in the Twentieth Century," *Milbank Memorial Fund Quarterly/Health and Society* 55 (Summer 1977):405-428.

21. J.P. Newhouse and M.J. Friedlander, *The Relationship Between Medical Resources and Measures of Health: Some Additional Evidence.* (Santa Monica, Calif.: The Rand Corporation, 1977), cited by Victor Fuchs, "Economics, Health, and Post-Industrial Society," *Milbank Memorial Fund Quarterly/Health and Society* 57 (Spring 1979):156.

22. Victor Fuchs, "Economics, Health, and Post-Industrial Society," *Milbank Memorial Fund Quarterly/Health and Society* 57 (Spring 1979):156.

23. See Frank Ackerman and Andrew Zimbalist, "Capitalism and Inequality in the United States," in Richard Edwards, Michael Reich, and Thomas Weisskopf, eds., *The Capitalist System*, 2nd ed. (Englewood Cliffs, N.J.: Prentice-Hall, 1978), pp. 293-307.

24. See M. Harvey Brenner, "Effects of Adverse Changes in the National Economy on Health," paper presented at the 103rd meeting of the American Public Health Association, Chicago, Ill., 18 November 1975, p. 2.

25. Vicente Navarro, "An Explanation of the Composition, Nature, and Functions of the Present Health Sector of the United States," in Vicente Navarro, *Medicine Under Capitalism* (New York: Neale Watson Academic, 1977), pp. 135-169.

26. Vicente Navarro, "The Underdevelopment of Health of Working America: Causes, Consequences and Possible Solutions," in Vicente Navarro, *Medicine Under Capitalism* (New York: Neale Watson Academic, 1977), pp. 82-99.

27. See Richard Auster, Irving Leveson, and Deborah Sarachek, "The Production of Health, an Exploratory Study," in Victor Fuchs, ed., *Essays in the Economics of Health and Medical Care* (New York: National Bureau of Economic Research, Columbia University Press, 1972), pp. 135-158; and Michael Grossman, "The Correlation Between Health and Schooling" in Nestor Terlecky, ed., *Household Production and Consumption* (New York: National Bureau of Economic Research, Columbia University Press, 1975), pp. 147-211.

28. Samuel Bowles, "Schooling and the Reproduction of Inequality," in Richard Edwards, Michael Reich, and Thomas Weisskopf, eds, *The Capitalist System*, 2nd ed. (Englewood Cliffs, N.J.: Prentice-Hall, 1978), p. 324. For a more extensive treatment of these ideas, see Samuel Bowles and Herbert Gintis, *Schooling in Capitalist America* (New York: Basic Books, 1976).

29. See Lester Lave and Eugene Seskin, *Air Pollution and Human Health* (Baltimore: The Johns Hopkins University Press, 1977), especially Appendix A.

30. See Leonard Gianessi et al., "The Distributional Effects of Uniform Air Pollution Policy in the United States," *Quarterly Journal of Economics* 93 (May 1979):281-301; and Richard England and Barry Bluestone, "Ecology and Social Conflict," in Herman Daly, ed., *Toward a Steady-State Economy* (San Francisco: Freeman, 1973), pp. 190-214.

31. For a discussion of the concept of the steady-state economy and its underlying assumptions, see Herman Daly, *Steady-State Economics* (San Francisco: Freeman, 1977), chap. 2.

10 Incentives for Quality in a Restructured Medical-Care System

Jon B. Christianson and
Walter McClure

Rising medical-care expenditures and the increasing proportion of those expenditures paid by government make inevitable some public-sector action to restructure the present medical-care-delivery system. In our view, there are two alternatives that hold the greatest promise for success in restraining expenditure increases in the future. One option is to give some (private or public) agency authority to set an areawide maximum limit on the annual allowable expenditures for a specified set of medical services; concommitantly, some (private or public) agency is given authority to implement a set of controls designed to keep expenditures within this limit. We refer to this method of expenditure containment as an "expenditure lid," or "lid-oriented regulatory system." A second option is to promote through appropriate public- and private-sector policies the widespread establishment of organized groups of providers that would compete for patients under fair-market conditions with traditional insurance plans and fee-for-service providers. These sets of providers would offer predetermined benefit packages at annual, per-capita rates. Examples of such organized groups include, but are by no means restricted to, Health Maintenance Organizations, Independent Practice Associations, Family Practice Plans, and Health Care Alliances. (For a description of several of these groups, see Enthoven 1978.) We refer to this option as the "competitive," or "market," approach to containing expenditures. (In addition to expenditure restraint, both of these options also can address the issues of access, equity, and coverage when combined with a compatible financing system. See McClure 1976.)

Either reform alternative must change the way in which physicians practice medicine if it is to be successful, ultimately, in restraining expenditure increases. That is, it must alter the manner in which particular procedures are performed and/or the mix of procedures that are provided for a given population. Thus either of these options, if effective, could have an impact on "quality of medical care," as it is commonly perceived. Identification of the incentives relating to quality of care that are implicit in both proposals is therefore a matter of interest for policymakers and medical-care analysts and is the primary objective of this chapter.

The authors gratefully acknowledge the financial support of the Hartford Foundation and the Bush Foundation.

121

Issues concerning quality of care are exceedingly complex. In the interests of brevity, we do not develop our arguments in great detail, instead substituting references for detailed exposition where possible and appropriate. Consequently, our discussion is primarily useful in suggesting lines of reasoning and raising important issues. The analysis we present is speculative rather than empirical. Since neither reform alternative has been implemented fully in the United States, data bearing directly on the questions of interest are limited. The results of quality-of-care studies in HMOs, for example, although positive (Williamson and Cunningham 1980) are not directly applicable to the analysis since the HMOs have not been subject to the extensive competition advocated by the competitive approach. Similarly, the performance of the British medical-care system provides only limited guidance to the outcomes of a lid-oriented regulatory system as it might evolve in the United States. However, we do review the experience of multiple HMOs competing for medicaid recipients in California for two reasons: the notoriety this experiment has received as an alleged example of "competitive" HMOs delivering poor-quality medical services, and the lessons that can be learned from the California experience concerning implementation of the competitive approach in a manner that would enhance quality of care. We begin by offering some general observations concerning the dimensions of quality in the delivery of medical care, followed by a discussion of the incentive changes under each reform as they would affect these dimensions.

The Concept of Quality

While there is certainly a social concensus concerning the desirability of high-quality medical care, there apparently is less of a consensus regarding the definition and measurement of that quality (Brook and Appel 1973; McClure 1973; McAuliffe 1979). We will use the term *microquality* when referring to the manner in which a physician responds to a patient's complaint. High-quality medical care in this sense means implementation of all diagnostic tests and treatment procedures that could reasonably be expected to improve the medical condition of the patient without undue risk. Under the present system of almost universal, comprehensive medical insurance, the existing incentives encourage the pursuit of microquality up to a point. The reimbursement system rewards the provider for doing more and therefore encourages the performance of all appropriate tests and procedures. But it also may encourage physicians to perform procedures for which they are not qualified, or which are of questionable relevance, but nevertheless are financially rewarding. To the extent that this occurs, the present system does not encourage microquality since it may result in the exposure of patients to undue risk. Furthermore, there are no inherent strong incentives in the present system that encourage peer review and consultation on the part of physicians. In our view, this type of peer interaction is an essential safeguard against inferior micro-quality in the delivery of medical care.

If resources were infinite, the quality of medical care for a given population could be maximized simply by assuring that appropriate procedures were performed in response to specific complaints. Unfortunately, the pursuit of quality is not an unconstrained maximization problem (Ellwood et al. 1973; Hiatt 1975). Since the resources that can, and will, be devoted to medical care by our society are finite, we must be concerned with what we term *"macroquality,"* or the utilization of available finite resources so as to attain the best possible health outcomes for a given population. One aspect of macroquality involves minimizing the waste of available medical resources by unnecessary duplication of tests and procedures. There are few incentives for the efficient management of individual patients, let alone defined populations, within the present medical-care system. Since no one provider is totally responsible for the care delivered to a particular patient, there is the potential for the performance of wasteful and duplicative procedures as the patient is passed from provider to provider. Furthermore, no one provider is held accountable for the ultimate health outcome of the patient. Provider linkages in the present system that would encourage the cost-effective treatment of individuals and establish account-ability are weak, and research has frequently found both cost and quality to suffer as a result (Brook and Appel 1973).

A second aspect of macroquality involves the broad allocation of resources to uses where they have the greatest impact on health outcomes. Here again, pursuit of quality in a micro sense may not lead to the best health outcomes for the population as a whole. For example, it may be more effective in terms of the health of the entire population to devote fewer resources to open-heart surgery and more to the follow-up of chronic hypertension. This does not mean that open-heart surgery is poor care but rather that, given finite resources, a healthier population can be achieved by the resource reallocation. Enthoven (1978), among others, has argued that costs in the present system are unnecessarily high relative to health outcomes achieved because the system lacks incentives for providers to allocate resources in ways that maximize health outcomes for each given population.

Both of the reform proposals mentioned have the potential to impose an effective financial constraint on providers and no doubt would alter provider behavior. However, they establish different structures and different sets of incentives relating to quality of care. In the following discussion, we speculate on the potential for each reform to (1) encourage peer consultation and inter-action, (2) establish provider linkages and accountability, and (3) reallocate medical resources in ways that maximize health outcomes in specific popula-tions. We consider these to be the key dimensions for judging the likely impact of reform proposals on quality of care.

An Expenditure-Lid Approach

Assuming that the medical-care system continues to be reimbursed by a mix of private and public third parties, a simple model of expenditure-lid regulation would require that government set a maximum limit on medical-care expenditures in each local area and then enforce each area's limit with a combination of controls on prices, utilization, physician supply, and capital accumulation (McClure 1979). Increases in the expenditure lid could be pegged to general economic indicators not specifically reflecting medical costs and input prices. This would make increases definable and easily explainable to the public and reduce the ability of producers to lobby for "exceptions" on a case-by-case basis. An expenditure lid would be meaningless in itself if actual expenditures were permitted to float up beyond the lid unchecked. To see that this does not happen, some regulatory agency would have to be established and provided with an adequate set of regulatory controls and, equally important, the incentive to use them effectively. If expenditures started to escalate unacceptably in a given area, the regulatory agency would be expected to cut allowable prices, tighten utilization review and/or constrain supply and capital sufficiently that expenditures did not exceed the lid. Such a strategy could be operated by any state, or it could be adopted for the entire nation by the federal government.

The expenditure-lid approach would establish a structure that could be utilized to reallocate medical-care resources in ways that would enhance macroquality. For instance, regulators could use lid-based price controls to establish a price schedule that would promote a mix of services conducive to improved health outcomes while at the same time enforcing the expenditure limit. As a hypothetical example to illustrate this possibility, consider an area with a well-enforced lid but with providers maldistributed within the area. Suppose providers are concentrated on delivering overelaborate services to one part of the population and neglect basic services to a different part of the population. In this case, macroquality could be improved through a reallocation of providers and services. Suppose the regulatory agency sets the prices of basic services at attractive levels and very specialized services at less attractive price levels. (Capital controls also could be selectively applied, but we ignore them in this example for the sake of simplicity.) Then any efficient provider could enter the area and find a ready practice in the underserved population (in the absence of regulatory entry controls). To remain within the expenditure lid, the regulatory agency would be forced to reduce prices for all services and providers in the area. Because of the nature of the price structure adopted, this action would squeeze net earnings on specialty services harder than net earnings on basic services. Efficient providers would begin to find basic services financially more attractive, specialty services less attractive, and would have an incentive to provide more basic services to the underserved population.

(Regulators presumably could continue such fine tuning on prices until they had achieved the desired balance between basic and specialty services.) By this process, macroquality could be enhanced.

Although a structure that could facilitate a desirable reallocation of resources clearly would exist under an expenditure lid, the potential for its successful implementation is in fact limited by political considerations. The establishment of an effective expenditure lid would be vigorously opposed by providers. The political price of the lid could well involve capitulation to providers on such issues as the determination of the relative prices that would exist in a lid-based system. Even without such an agreement, the political bargaining that would inevitably surround the specification of relative prices would not be characterized by the balanced representation of diverse views. Providers would pursue their concentrated interests in lobbying the regulatory agency to specify a price schedule that generated more attractive earnings for highly specialized services than for basic services (Marmor, Wittman, and Heagy 1976; Noll 1975). Such a price schedule is more likely to reward providers for offering overelaborate care to professionally interesting patients rather than increased amounts of basic services for the entire area; thus it would skew the distribution of medical-care resources toward uses that were not cost effective and therefore were detrimental to macroquality. In opposition to these concentrated provider interests would be the relatively diffuse interests of the constituencies supportive of, for example, health promotion, health education, early prenatal care, and home care. Consequently, the process of defining a desirable balance between basic and specialized services (or among any types of services) and a price schedule with the incentives to promote that balance would be extremely vulnerable to special-interest pressures applied by providers.

The potential for improved provider linkages, accountability, and peer consultation under an expenditure lid seems equally limited. Again the accompanying regulatory apparatus could be used to establish a structure conducive to quality improvement. The present Professional Standards Review Organizations, for instance, could be expanded and increased in sophistication. However, this type of structure would not alter the underlying incentives of providers. The rewards to the physician for engaging in serious peer consultation or patient follow-up likely would be low relative to the marginal benefits of devoting the same time and effort to lobbying for desirable regulatory rulings or, at the least, for rulings that would not alter existing practice patterns.

In summary, the appeal of the expenditure-lid approach is its potential for establishing a structure of prices and controls that could arguably improve quality. However, the actual development and implementation of any quality-improvement mechanisms would take place in a highly politicized process and would meet with substantial opposition on the part of concentrated provider interests. Therefore, the reality of quality in an expenditure-lid system likely would fall considerably short of its potential.

A Competitive Approach

Competition in the delivery of medical services can be increased by creating sets of providers among whom consumers can choose for care such that the premium paid by each consumer reflects the efficiency of the providers chosen (McClure 1978; Christianson and McClure 1980). (We will refer to these sets of providers as "health-care plans," a generic term that includes the Health Maintenance Organization but is broad enough to encompass many other organizational forms as well (McClure 1978). These health-care plans would be differentiated from traditional health-insurance plans since they would actually provide care. The most important feature of the plans for the stimulation of competition would be the circle they draw around specific sets of physicians and hospitals, with a separate premium for each.

Employees, medicare and medicaid recipients, and all other individuals would be offered a choice among these plans. However, it is likely that the majority of enrollment decisions would continue to occur at the worksite. Employers would play a major role in selecting health-care plans and traditional insurance plans as benefit options and would supervise the actual enrollment process. Each employee would receive a fixed dollar contribution from the employer for whichever option was selected. The employee would be required to pay (or, if negative, would receive) the difference between this contribution and the plan premium.

Competition among health-care plans and traditional insurance plans would have the effect of experience-rating providers. Incentives would be created for providers to be conscious of expenditures since their ability to secure and retain a patient population would depend in part on the competitiveness of their premiums. Consumers would have an incentive to be cost conscious since they would have a financial stake in the choice of health-benefit option. (This contrasts with the present system of medical-care reimbursement where there is little reward for consumers who choose efficient providers or for providers who practice cost-effective medicine.) Under a competitive system, expenditures on medical services probably would continue to increase, but the degree of expenditure containment achieved probably would be similar to that of a well-enforced expenditure lid tied to general economic indicators. However, the nature of the expenditure-containment mechanism would be quite different. Under a competitive system providers would choose the mix of cost-effective medical practices they desired, subject to the necessity of attracting consumers. Under an expenditure lid, they would adopt these practices in response to regulatory decrees or as an adaptation to regulated fee schedules, if at all. It is this distinction that also results in different sets of incentives for quality under the two reform proposals.

When operating effectively, a competitive system featuring multiple health-care plans would contain incentives for an improved allocation of resources. Under such a system providers would not be able to finance ineffective resource allocations or overlapping and inefficient treatment regimens through the cost-plus reimbursement system that presently exists, or through the exercise of political power that appears possible under an expenditure lid. Plans adopting expensive, unproven technology or practicing overelaborate medicine would have high premiums and presumably low enrollments. Thus in a competitive system, successful plans would find it in their own best interest to identify and implement simple, relatively low-cost, primary-care measures with high probabilities of improving the health of their enrolled membership. If a specific measure implemented by one plan were found to be effective, it would be adopted quickly by other health-care plans as well. Health-care plans that did not seek out such innovations would be at a premium disadvantage in attracting enrollees. Thus the competitive system would reward flexibility and innovation in the delivery of medical care.

It also seems probable that health care outcomes would be easier to measure and monitor in a competitive system. In a health-care plan, the accountability of a defined set of providers for the health-care needs of a defined set of consumers is established, in contrast with the current system that holds providers accountable only for particular patient episodes. For example, if low rates of child immunization and relatively high rates of disease prevalence occur in a population at present, no provider is held accountable for this failure nor is any responsible to correct it. If the membership of a health-care plan exhibited similar characteristics, plan providers clearly would be held accountable. This accountability and the professional ethics of providers are the consumer's primary safeguards against skimping and underservice in a competitive system. (Furthermore, in a competitive-environment health-care plan they might find it to their advantage to monitor the performance of their competitors and question any abnormal health outcomes they might observe.) Since health-care plans would market their services in part by emphasizing their record of performance, information on health outcomes associated with particular providers would become available to employers and potential enrollees, and these groups would become more sophisticated in evaluating provider performance. Therefore it seems likely that competition among health-care plans for members would increase the quality consciousness of purchasers of medical services.

Finally, this type of competition would create incentives for the development of quality-assurance systems on the part of providers. Health-care plans, by their organizational structure, would facilitate and legitimize peer consultation and review. Unlike the present system (or an expenditure-lid system) where peer review is an onerous policing duty that can alienate referral sources, in a competitive system physicians participating in health-care plans would want to assure that their colleagues were practicing medicine of acceptable quality that would not discredit the plan to employers and enrollees. If a plan were to acquire a reputation for poor-quality care, its enrollment presumably would suffer.

In summary, the appeal of the competitive approach is that if an effective competitive structure could be established, providers would find it in their own interest to adopt procedures that assured quality in both a macro and a micro-sense. However, the reality of quality in a competitive system would depend on the degree to which providers could be kept in a truly competitive environment, with multiple health-care plans competing for the attention of informed employers and consumers. If health-care plans were able to successfully segment the medical-care marketplace, or in some other way avoid direct competitive pressures, the potential incentives for resource reallocation and peer review under the competitive approach would be reduced. The potential for improved quality in a competitive system also would be diminished of incentives for careful evaluation if health-care plans by employers and consumers were weak.

Learning from Medi-Cal

In the early 1970s the state of California encouraged the development of health-care plans to provide medical services to the poor under the auspices of its medicaid program (Medi-Cal). The plans negotiated contracts with the state for the nonexclusive right to enroll Medi-Cal eligibles. In return, the health-care plans received a fixed monthly premium per enrollee that was set at least 10 percent below the per-capita costs of fee-for-service care. The fixed-payment arrangement was intended to reduce incentives for costly "overprovision" of services to medicaid recipients and to stimulate further efficiencies through competition among the plans.

By 1973 approximately 250,000 Medi-Cal eligibles were enrolled in 55 HMOs. A large proportion of these HMOs were formed specifically to serve California Medi-Cal eligibles, and the majority of their enrollees were from this group. By all accounts, the results of this experiment were extremely negative (Goldberg 1975; Lewis, Fein, and Mechanic 1976; Spitz 1979). As Spitz observes, there were "indications of gross underutilization of services. . . denials of emergency care and poor treatment" (Spitz 1979, p. 512). An apparently large proportion of medicaid payments were used for "administration" as opposed to patient treatment (Lewis, Fein, and Mechanic 1976).

As other authors have noted, there were numerous unique aspects of the Medi-Cal experience that make it difficult to generalize from the results (Goldberg 1975; Spitz 1979). However, there do seem to be (at least) two major differences in the Medi-Cal program and the competitive approach described above that result in different incentives with respect to quality of care.

Nature of the Enrolled Group: Employees versus
Medicaid Recipients

Auger and Goldberg (1974) point out that three primary constraints on under-service by competitive health-care plans—the medical ethics of physicians, the threat of malpractice suits, and the potential for incurrence of future costs—all are weaker when treating a patient population consisting of medicaid receipients as opposed to employed groups. For example, a physician's ethical code is likely to have the strongest restraining influence when dealing with patients of his own social class. On the other hand, it promises to be the least effective with respect to welfare recipients, particularly when poverty is complicated by racial differences.

The threat of a malpractice suit also is reduced when treating medicaid recipients. Medi-Cal recipients seldom entered into malpractice suits, presumably because of income restraints, ignorance of the legal resources available to them, or intimidation by the legal system (Goldberg 1975). The inclination of middle-class, employed individuals to seek legal recourse presumably would be much greater.

Third, Goldberg (1975) points out that health-care plans may be less concerned with the future costs of underservice to present enrollees if they do not expect to bear these costs. Since the turnover in medicaid programs is usually quite high (Spitz 1979), this seems a reasonable expectation for health-care plans serving primarily Medi-Cal enrollees. However, the relative stability of the workforce for most private employers would make this a less reasonable expectation in a competitive system such as described earlier.

Another important difference between Medi-Cal eligibles and employed groups relates to the financial obligation of enrollees. In the competitive approach, the employee typically would have a financial stake in the enrollment decision. This provides an additional incentive to carefully evaluate available health-care plans. In contrast, Medi-Cal covered the full premium for whichever option was chosen by the medicaid eligible. From an equity point of view this policy was judged to be desirable, but it probably reduced the perceived benefits to the enrollees of carefully evaluating all options.

Performance of the "Middleman": Employers versus
Medicaid Agencies

Spitz (1979) found that medicaid agencies exerted little effective influence on the performance of health-care plans in California. This conclusion contrasts with the active role that many employers have played in the monitoring and evaluation of HMOs in other areas (Christianson and McClure 1979). Employers have a strong incentive to be careful in the selection of the health-care plans that they offer to employees in order to minimize subsequent employee dissatisfaction with their health-care benefits. Therefore they often conduct extensive evaluation of health-care plans that go beyond superficial examinations of benefit coverage and premiums to the selective auditing of health-care-plan medical records. Consequently, when health-care plans are offered as benefit options, they already have passed a relatively thorough "quality check." Although medicaid agencies theoretically perform a similar role for eligibles, they appear to be less effective, possibly due to political pressures and budget limitations.

After offering health-care plans, employers continue to monitor their performance and assess employee satisfaction with medical care provided by the plans (Christianson and McClure 1979). This assessment generally takes the form of periodic surveys of employees who are members of health-care plans. When problems are identified, the employer plays an active role in negotiating with the health-care plan to improve service. Again, while government agencies could function in a similar manner with respect to medicaid eligibles, they face legal and procedural restrictions that limit their ability to discipline health-care plans that perform poorly (Spitz 1979).

In summary, the characteristics of the medicaid population and the apparent limitations on the effectiveness of state government performance as a "middleman" appear to have contributed to the poor-quality care provided by many HMOs in the early stages of the Medi-Cal program. Neither of these factors would be present in the competitive approach described in this chapter. The Medi-Cal experience underscores the importance for quality of care of instituting the competitive reform first with the employed middle class. Health-care plans that satisfy the scrutiny of these buyers then could be offered to the medicaid population with a high degree of confidence.

Summary and Conclusions

Both reform proposals—the expenditure lid and the competitive approach—promise to restrain expenditure increases for medical services. Each could potentially alter provider behavior and therefore affect quality of care. The expenditure-lid approach has a surface appeal since it contains regulatory mechanisms that could be used to improve quality. A closer examination indicates that there are severe political limitations on the effective use of these regulatory tools. If the potential of the expenditure-lid approach with respect to improving quality of care is to be realized, the concentrated interests of providers in the political arena must be counterbalanced in some way.

In contrast, the competitive approach would seem, on the surface, to invite the underprovision of services. However, on more careful consideration, an effective competitive market would appear to contain strong provider incentives for the enhancement of quality. For the potential of the competitive approach to be developed, means must be found to establish competitive health-care plans on a large scale and to ensure that competitive incentives are maintained on a continuing basis in markets where health-care plans exist. In this regard, implementation of the competitive reform first in the employed middle class would seem appropriate.

The speculative nature of the analysis cautions against drawing strong conclusions. However, the quality-of-care issues that we have raised in this chapter certainly deserve careful consideration in the future by those policymakers and medical-care analysts who support either expenditure lids or competitive markets as cost-containment methods.

References

Auger, Richard C., and Goldberg, Victor P. 1974. "Prepaid Health Plans and Moral Hazard," *Public Policy* 22 (No. 3) (Summer):353-397.

Brook, Robert H., and Appel, Francis A. 1973. "Quality-of-Care Assessment: Choosing a Method for Peer Review," *New England Journal of Medicine* 288 (No. 25) (June 21):1323-1329.

Christianson, Jon B., and McClure, Walter. 1980. "Developing a Regulatory Strategy Consistent with a Competitive Medical Care System," *Socioeconomic Issues of Health 1980*, Douglas Hough, ed., Center for Health Services Research and Development, American Medical Association, forthcoming.

Christianson, Jon B., and McClure, Walter. 1979. "Competition in the Delivery of Medical Care," *New England Journal of Medicine* 301 (No. 15) (October 11):812-818.

Ellwood, Paul M., O'Donoghue, Patrick, McClure, Walter, Holley, Robert, Carlson, Rick J., and Hoagberg, Earl. 1973. *Assuring the Quality of Health Care*. Minneapolis: InterStudy.

Enthoven, Alain C. 1978. "Shattuck Lecture: Cutting Cost Without Cutting the Quality of Care," *New England Journal of Medicine* 298 (No. 22) (June 1):1229-1238.

Goldberg, Victor P. 1975. "Some Emerging Problems of Prepaid Health Plans in the Medi-Cal System," *Policy Analysis* 1 (No. 1) (Winter):55-68.

Hiatt, Howard H. 1975. "Protecting the Medical Commons: Who Is Responsible?" *New England Journal of Medicine* 293 (No. 5) (July 31):235-241.

Lewis, Charles E., Fein, Rashi, and Mechanic, David. 1976. *A Right to Health: The Problem of Access to Primary Medical Care*. New York: Wiley, pp. 235-237.

Marmor, Theodore, Wittman, Donald, and Heagy, Thomas. 1976. "The Politics of Medical Inflation," *Journal of Health Politics, Policy and Law* 1 (No. 1) (Spring):69-84.

McAuliffe, William E. 1979. "Measuring the Quality of Medical Care: Process Versus Outcome," *Milbank Memorial Fund Quarterly/Health and Society* 57 (No. 1) (Winter):118-152.

McClure, Walter. 1979. *Comprehensive Market and Regulatory Strategies for Medical Care*, report prepared for Bureau of Health Planning and Resource Development, DHEW, Contract Number HRA-230-77-033 (April 9).

_____. 1973. "Four Points on Quality Assurance," *Quality Assurance of Medical Care*, edited by Regional Medical Programs Service, Washington, D.C. Health Services and Mental Health Administration, DHEW.

_____. 1976. "The Medical Care System under National Health Insurance: Four Models," *Journal of Health Policy, Politics, and Law* 1 (No. 1) (Spring):22-68.

_____. 1978. "On Broadening the Definition of and Removing Regulatory Barriers to a Competitive Health Care System," *Journal of Health Policy, Politics, and Law* 3 (No. 3) (Fall):303-327.

Noll, Roger. 1975. "The Consequences of Public Utility Regulation of Hospitals," *Controls on Health Care.* Washington, D.C.: Institute of Medicine, National Academy of Sciences, pp. 25-48.

Spitz, Bruce. 1979. "When a Solution Is Not a Solution: Medicaid and Health Maintenance Organizations," *Journal of Health Politics, Policy and Law* 3 (No. 4) (Winter):497-518.

Williamson, J., and Cunningham, F. 1980. "How Does Quality of Care in HMOs Compare?" *Group Health Journal* (Winter):4-25.

**Part V
Comparative Health Issues**

11 Drawing Lessons from Comparative Health Research

Deborah A. Stone

Comparative health-policy research is a field characterized by the optimism of its researchers in the face of strong pessimism among its users. People engage in comparative research largely because they believe that it is possible to learn useful lessons from other countries and that such learning put into practice will ultimately improve the human condition. If the amount of money spent on comparative health research, or the number of publications in the field, are any indicators of belief in the value of cross-national studies, then one would have to say that the field has certainly been flourishing. On the other hand, considering the vast volume of comparative health research that is produced, one is hard pressed to point to specific instances of the *use* of lessons from research in health-policy practice.

While everyone believes that we ought to be able to learn from abroad, very few comparative studies make the leap from description and analysis of foreign health systems to a statement of lessons for health policymakers. The field has yet to overcome some critical obstacles.

Barriers to Learning from Abroad

The Assumption of Uniqueness

Perhaps the most serious obstacle to learning from abroad is the pervasive feeling among Americans (and probably other nationals too) that "our country is unique." American individualistic values, translated onto a national scale, lead to a belief that all countries are different, as though they have different personalities, and that policies for different countries must therefore have separate origins. Discussions of comparative health systems (or of any comparative public-policy studies, for that matter) are peppered with phrases about the "unique historical experiences," "different pattern of development," "different cultural values," "different social customs," "different popular attitudes" that characterize different nations.

Ideas gleaned from abroad are often greeted with the pronouncement that "they would not work here," backed up by an explanation that they would not

I would like to thank Mark Segal for his research assistance in this chapter.

work because of our unique history, development, culture, social customs, or attitudes. To some extent, this concern with national differences is a valid recognition of the fact that health systems are embedded in specific historical and political contexts and cannot simply be extracted and transplanted. But too often such recitations of the differences among countries are used as glib excuses for refusing to delve more deeply and with an open mind into the practices of another country.

The assumption of uniqueness is backed by arguments that have great intuitive appeal but are very hard to test. It is very hard to argue against claims that a system or program works in a foreign country because the citizens have certain "attitudes," "traditions," "tastes," or "habits." (It would also be hard to show in a positive sense that such attitudes and so on actually exist.) Moreover, there is a very important hidden assumption behind the uniqueness argument, namely, that culture (attitudes, tastes, traditions, habits, customs, values, and so on) is a *given* in any society and is impossible to change. Therefore policymakers have no control over these factors and may as well not make futile efforts to alter them. To argue that a system or program works abroad because of the nation's culture is to absolve oneself of any responsibility to try the idea in one's own country. At the very least, the researcher or analyst ought to attempt to isolate the precise connection between a belief (attitude, value, and so on) and the policy result it is alleged to cause or enable.

The Assumption that Learning Means Copying

Very much related to the assumption that all countries are unique and therefore unable to learn from one another is the assumption that the only kind of learning involves copying the system in use in another country. The possibility of learning from abroad is dismissed, with the explanation that "we can not adopt their system because we are different." Underneath this assumption lie both a valid lesson and a fallacy.

The valid lesson, learned from many instances of attempted export of American health practices and technologies, is that no matter how simple, efficacious, and obviously beneficial some innocation seems, it may not be adopted wholeheartedly by the people whom it would allegedly benefit, and its transfer to a foreign country or culture may lead to many unintended consequences. The literature of public health is replete with studies attempting to determine why the gifts of health practices and systems from advanced countries to less developed, or from colonizing countries to their colonies, were not incorporated into local practices (Elling 1980, p. 87). Perhaps some of our reluctance to believe we can learn from abroad comes from our experience in trying to *teach* and impart our knowledge in other nations.

The fallacy underlying this assumption, however, is the implicit notion that the only kind of learning is direct imitation or direct transfer of foreign practices. In fact, there are many ways one can learn from abroad and put those lessons into practice, besides wholesale borrowing. At the very least, one can learn from another country's failures and thereby learn what not to adopt. But in between the endpoints of incomplete imitation and complete rejection lies a whole spectrum of types of learning. These are explored in the second half of this chapter.

The Assumption of Individual Determinism

One very strong current in comparative research is the classical-liberal assumption that individual decision making is the motor that drives the health system. That the market metaphor should be used in comparative research is not very surprising since so much of the analysis of domestic health policy is predicated on the assumption of a market for health services. In comparative studies, much effort has been devoted to explaining why individuals do and do not adopt medical innovations introduced from outside their culture.

Early interest in health-care practices of nonwesternized peoples grew out of the desires of public-health officials to introduce certain preventive health-care measures such as sanitary disposal of human and animal wastes, water purification, and healthy nutrition. Even today, the largest cross-national study of health services, which covered twelve locations in seven countries and took years to complete, is a study of "health-care utilization" (Kohn and White 1976). Research on utilization takes the individual as the unit of analysis and tries to explain why he or she decides to use particular medical services in much the same way as market researchers try to determine what makes an individual buy a certain product.

While most health-policy analysts would agree that individual decision making does play a role in determining who gets what care, comparative health research has probably placed too heavy an emphasis on this approach. The focus on individual decisions about using health services to explain the success or failure of health systems ignores (or at least downplays) the role of collective decisions and government policy. More important, the emphasis of comparative health research on individual attitudes and practices has had two adverse consequences for lesson drawing.

First, the knowledge base in the field of comparative health systems is heavily slanted toward a knowledge of individual health practices and attitudes. The researcher looking for a simple description of the organization of health services in a foreign country (particularly a lesser developed country) may often find a wealth of information on the quaint practices of exotic tribes and cultures but no overall description of health care as a social and political institution. If the only knowledge to be gleaned from foreign countries is an understanding of the health beliefs and practices of its inhabitants, there is not much reason for drawing lessons for one's own country. Possible lessons about the organization, financing, administration, regulation of health services will be largely ignored.

Secondly, to the extent that researchers think that a health system is shaped primarily by the attitudes and choices of its individual users, they will see little hope for transforming the system through more centralized policy decisions. Thus they will be less likely to *look* for lessons that will be useful to policymakers.

The Assumption of the Contaminated Source

It has been well established in the fields of social psychology and public opinion that the readiness of individuals to believe new information is strongly affected by their relationship to the source from which they learn the information. Information is more readily accepted from people who are perceived as authority figures and who are thought to share important values.

An analogous phenomenon can be observed on the national scale. In looking abroad for lessons for our health-care system, we are most apt to look at countries whose political systems and ideology are most like our own. Thus we look to countries whose political system is democratic, whose economies are based on private ownership and entrepreneurship, and whose cultures put strong value on individual achievement and freedom of individual choice. There is sometimes an implicit assumption in health-policy discussions that if we borrow lessons from the health-care system of a country whose political and ideological stances we do not share, we will be introducing a contaminant into our own system, and the new health innovation will have very disruptive consequences for society.

The best examples of this assumption in American health-policy debates concern efforts to introduce national health insurance in the United States. Between 1915 and 1920, when national health insurance came into the policy agenda for the first time, a major source of opposition was the historical fact that the first national health insurance program had been created by Bismarck during the imperial regime of William II and that the Soviet Union had adopted national health insurance. Many people argued that national health insurance was then inextricably tied to monarchism or socialism and thus was inappropriate in a democratic republic. Opponents denounced compulsory health insurance as "made in Germany," "European paternalism run mad," and "infamous Kultur imported to this country by a Russian disciple of Bolshevism and I-won't-workism" (Lubove 1968, pp. 82-90). When national health insurance was again debated during the 1940s and 1950s, the American Medical Association launched a major public-education campaign and lobbying effort against it. The thrust of the campaign was the argument that national health insurance constituted "socialized medicine" and that its supporters were left-wing organizations, radicals, and members of the Communist Party. To allow national health insurance would lead to "socialization of other phases of American life" (Harris 1966, pp. 27-47).

To the extent that policymakers are influenced by the image of a contaminated source of knowledge, one would expect there to be a certain heirarchy of knowledge that is accepted from abroad. Policymakers would be most receptive to knowledge that is perceived as "purely technical" and least receptive to that perceived as political or social. Acceptance of knowledge from technical fields, or technical innovation, is usually thought to have limited repercussions. Social and political consequences are not often forseen so that the importation of technical knowledge is rarely opposed on grounds that it might lead to political disruption. The more the knowledge is perceived as *directly* linked to social and political organization, the more its potential side-effects will be invoked as a barrier to importation or adoption.

In the field of medical care and health policy, one could probably designate a hierarchy of subfields according to whether they are perceived as more technical or more political. Clinical knowledge (the understanding of treatment of individual cases) is probably perceived as less political than epidemiological knowledge (the understanding of disease processes in large groups), and epidemiological knowledge as less political than policy knowledge (the understanding of the organization, financing, and control of the health-care system). One would then expect to find the most cross-national transfer of knowledge in clinical medicine, less in epidemiology, and least in health-systems organization, financing, and control.

But this is not to argue that clinical and epidemiological knowledge are not political. One can find many examples of a nation refusing to accept knowledge of either kind for political reasons. A notable example in the United States is the refusal of the Food and Drug Administration to accept some data from drug tests performed abroad. Until 1975 foreign research could not be used to support a new drug application (the so-called NDA). And new drugs are still required to undergo certain testing in the United States before they may be certified, even though the shunning of foreign tests has apparently contributed to a significant drug lag (U.S. Government Accounting Office 1980).

Epidemics, because they are almost by definition a wide-scale social problem, are potentially dangerous politically.

Like riots, famines, wars, fires, mass strikes and rebellions, epidemics are stages for collective self-recognition and for the reconstruction of collective identities normally subordinated in every day life to publicly acceptable "roles." (Stark 1977, p. 687)

Governments are often reluctant to "declare" epidemics because declarations constitute an admission of crisis and put pressure on the state to solve the problem. In the United States, we are currently witnessing this phenomenon with respect to the "Agent Orange" syndrome. Veterans groups are trying to establish that a wide variety of symptoms experienced by people who have been exposed to Agent Orange (a chemical defoliant used in Vietnam) are in fact a related syndrome and thus, that there is an epidemic. The Veterans Administration is resisting their claims and maintains the position that there is little evidence to show an epidemic, for which, incidentally, the U.S. government could be held responsible. Internationally, there are many other examples of cover-ups of epidemics. And when governments are anxious to conceal epidemics, they will certainly be unreceptive to having their epidemics studied or to sharing their own knowledge with other countries.

Practical Barriers to Learning

The four assumptions explored are all habits of thinking that prevent people from learning as much as possible from knowledge gleaned through comparative research. One should also mention, however, a less ethereal reason why we rarely draw lessons from comparative research: the extraordinary difficulty of doing comparative research in the first place.

Granted that comparative research is fun and that the people who engage in it probably have a taste for travel, the difficulties of producing valid research that has scientific respectability are enormous. Travel to foreign sites is expensive. The researcher must usually learn at least one foreign language, and even then, communication can be difficult. If the research requires living abroad for any length of time, the researcher must establish a home, learn to shop in a new place, establish a social network and learn new social customs, and establish a professional network. (Some of these considerations are described by William Glaser 1977, who has conducted several multicountry studies.)

Any cross-national study presents a significant research-design problem. The major challenge to the research is to define concepts within the health system that are comparable in different nations. Even the simple problem of comparing health resources across nations is very complex. Should we simply count the doctor/population ratio? If so, does one count medical students and doctors in training? They are probably allowed to perform very different tasks in different countries so that they are not a "standardized" measure of service. Even fully licensed doctors in countries with relatively similar medical systems may provide very different levels and types of care. In West Germany, for example, specialists may not provide primary care (as specialists may in the United States), hospital-based physicians may not provide ambulatory care (with a few exceptions), and occupational physicans may not provide primary care. Thus simply counting heads does not give us a very accurate picture of the actual services available to a population.

The problem is even more vivid when one trys to compare the number of hospital beds across countries:

> What is a bed? It may be a rope stretched between the sides of a wooden frame, or it may be canvas with no sheets or blankets. It may have a mattress and sheets but may be attended only by auxiliary personnel; or doctors and nurses may be there, but a lack of equipment and materials may seriously limit the quality of service. These differences are seen between countries and within a country, and they may be the differences between the last century and this century in terms of medical care. (Bryant 1969, p. 49)

Although the researcher may want (or need) to rely on official statistics for a basic description of national health systems, the categories may be defined very differently by different national agencies. Thus, for example, in data on infant mortality, France counts a birth as "live" only after the baby has lived 24 hours, while most other countries begin counting from the moment of birth. George Myers (1976) has explored the ramifications of this and numerous other factors for the reliability of infant-mortality statistics. Yet infant-mortality and adulty-mortality rates are generally considered the most reliable (if not very informative) cross-national measures of health status.

An excellent discussion of the difficulties of cross-national studies of health systems is provided by Ray Elling (1980). Without going into a lengthy discussion here, the point to be made is that *learning* from cross-national research is doubly difficult because simply *conducting* the research is also difficult.

Types of Lessons

It is possible to learn many kinds of lessons from cross-national health research, as was so ably shown by Marmor, Bridges, and Bickart (1980). The following outline follows essentially their discussion of five types of learning: stretching the range of policy considerations, weighing the determinants of policy, evaluating new policy options, understanding the impact of institutional structure on policy implementation.

Generating Ideas for Program Design

If comparative research can do nothing else, it can provide policymakers with a range of different solutions to problems encountered by several countries. In the field of health policy, cross-national studies can illustrate myriad administrative and financial arrangements for health insurance and for the regulation of cost and quality of services. Comparative research for the purposes of yielding new ideas is somewhat akin to going on an international shopping spree. The research design does not need to be sophisticated in order to gather ideas.

Research for the purposes of generating new ideas has both advantages and disadvantages. On the plus side, truly creative new ideas are hard to come by so that casting a wide net in the search of innovative solutions is the best possible technique. People have certain "cultural blocks" that make particular solutions or ideas unthinkable (Adams 1974, pp. 31-47). Ideas that might be dismissed by colleagues as "foolhardy" or "irresponsible" in one country might be already in use with effective results in another country. Cross-national research can help expand our notions of what is possible and acceptable.

The disadvantage of idea-generating research is that this type is most often dismissed as inapplicable. The gathering of a grocery cart full of solutions from abroad is often greeted with the assumption of uniqueness: "We are different from them" and "it will not work here." Without more careful analysis of the efficacy of individual options in their own national context and of the factors that determine efficacy, policymakers are reluctant to take the ideas very seriously. Even when researchers provide more sophisticated analyses of a foreign program, policymakers and politicians may still dismiss the idea as unworkable with claims that the "culture" (or "tastes," "traditions," "attitudes," or "habits") of the foreign nation is the true explanation for why the idea works abroad.

An example of this phenomenon is seen in American analyses of Swedish hospital-staffing patterns. In 1959 Paul Lembcke reported that Swedish hospitals use only about half the personnel per patient as American hospitals with no apparent difference in outcomes for patients or quality of care. But his work was widely criticized for its failure to control important variables such as severity of illness of patients, case, and length of stay. Nearly twenty years later, Jonsson and Neuhauser replicated Lembcke's findings with a more careful research design and then sought to explain the difference. But even the researchers themselves tended to look to ambiguous cultural factors for explaining their results rather than to political (and thus more controllable) factors. They suggested that a different work ethic among Swedish workers makes them work harder than their American counterparts; different tastes among Swedish patients make them demand fewer services of hospital personnel; and different political values make Swedish patients resistant to certain billing (and presumably thus hospital financing) arrangements. The authors conclude rather pessimistically that any small changes in hospital-staffing patterns (for example, reducing diagnostic work-up in U.S. hospitals) "might mean changing malpractice mechanisms at the institutional level, and this in turn may relate to macro-cultural values of justice and equity" (Jonsson and Neuhauser 1975, p. 136).

Understanding Causal Factors

One of the major thrusts of comparative health-policy research has been the attempt to explain why particular configurations of health systems developed in different countries. Such studies quite reasonably focus on historical develop-ment of health systems. But most studies of historical development have not been designed for the purposes of lesson drawing, and they are generally of more academic than policy interest.

Historical studies can be useful but only insofar as they distinguish the manipulable from the nonmanipulable factors of causation. To the extent that the modern configuration of health services is attributed to historical factors (for example, wars, revolutions) or situational events (for example, natural disasters, the charisma of specific leaders), the explanations will contain little usable information for policymakers. If researchers wish to draw lessons from historical research, they must carefully delineate the areas of human choice in the evolution of a health system. Even though a war may have been an impor-tant factor in shaping a health system (as the Boer Wars are said to be in the case of the British National Health Insurance), the researcher should inquire further into the human responses to the war. How were the choices perceived? How did the war lead people to consider some alternatives and not others? How did the experience of the war make the choice of one alternative more attractive? How did the wartime situation affect the political feasibility of the different alternatives? And finally, in what ways might policymakers create or avoid similar conditions if they want to adopt a policy choice similar to or different from the one under analysis.

To conduct analyses of causal factors, various scholars of comparative health policy have proposed three different types of research design. In the most-similar-systems design (Przeworski and Tuene 1970; Marmor, Bridges, and Bickart 1980), one starts with some ideas about the factors that ought plausibly to determine the nature of the health system and then searches for pairs or groups of countries that are alike on as many as possible of these dimensions. Theoretically, any observed differences in the health system are then attributable to other factors, that is, to dimensions on which the countries differ.

A variant of this approach, "contrasting pairs," (Elling 1980, pp. 63-64) suggests starting with well-known relationships in health policy and looking for deviant cases. For example, starting with the correlation between GNP per capita and infant-mortality rates, one would search for pairs of countries with similar infant-mortality rates but vastly different resource levels, or for pairs of countries where the relationship goes in the opposite direction. Such a study would lead one to examine the nonobvious causal factors and to examine the conditions under which secondary or weaker causal factors become dominant.

A third approach might be called the "evolutionary" or "developmental" approach. Rather than constructing a quasi-experimental design, scholars using this approach look for long-term historical trends in several nations and use these trends to predict how the health systems of other nations will evolve. This approach entails a deterministic view of history, and though it has more often been associated with Marxist analyses, one can find assertions of world-wide trends in the works of a range of scholars. Elling (1980, pp. 215-223) suggests that the health systems of colonized nations will undergo similar transformations as the societies are liberated. He explores how "modern" medicine is used to assist the colonizing country in taking over, maintaining colonial authority, "cooling out" opposition, and controlling the native population. Relationships and conflicts between modern and traditional medicine will parallel the political relationships between colonial and native forces.

Milton Roemer (1977), in the most comprehensive overview of comparative health policy yet published, concludes with an enumeration of worldwide trends that presumably apply to all countries, regardless of their economic and political organization. The trends include an increase in the supply of doctors and allied health personnel relative to population, increasing relative expenditures on health combined with increased concern for expenditure control, and increased emphasis on preventive care and health planning. Such general statements have greater descriptive than predictive or explanatory value, and in the end, may only illustrate Alford's claim (1976) that the rhetoric of health-policy reforms is only a reflection of efforts by established powerful groups to preserve their power.

Predicting the Impact of Policy Options

Comparative research is often said to create the opportunity for "natural experiments." The researcher can identify pairs or groups of countries judiciously so as to eliminate logically certain variables as causal factors. Or, alternatively, the researcher can choose countries with similar administrative or financial arrangements and to observe whether the arrangements produce similar results. As Marmor, Bridges, and Bickart (1980) and others have noted, no cross-national research is truly an experiment in the rigorous scientific sense, but this does not mean we should despair of learning from comparative research.

All health systems must respond to certain key problems—assuring access to services, maintaining quality of services, and controlling the costs of services—though the relative emphasis and the standards of success of these goals may differ. Likewise, all health systems must perform certain basic tasks; they must train or import health-care personnel, construct and maintain facilities, manufacture or import equipment and drugs, and control epidemics. By explaining (or describing) how different countries attempt to solve their basic problems and perform their basic tasks, comparative researchers can contribute to a general stock of knowledge about the impact of specific design features.

The experiences of other countries can provide usable information on a variety of questions. For example, what will be the impact of the introduction (or reduction) of cost sharing on patient behavior? How does physician behavior change when reimbursement methods or rates are changed? How does public opinion respond to physician strikes? Additionally, it would be useful to know what ideas have been tried and abandoned in other countries. For example, sickness funds in West Germany experimented with a cash bonus for members who did not visit a physician in a three-month period but discontinued the program as ineffective in saving costs. The sickness fund also shifted away from a fixed-budgeting system to fee-for-service reimbursement of physicians, but later found it desirable to reintroduce fixed budgeting (Stone 1979).

Understanding Political and Strategic Factors

Some interesting research in comparative health policy has focused on explaining what motivates and enables governments to enact certain policy reforms. This research has a very high potential for lesson drawing and is in fact often motivated by a desire to understand the range of politically feasible options. The work of Theodore Marmor and his associates has been pivotal in this field (Marmor and Thomas 1971 and 1972; Marmor, Whittman, and Heagy 1976). More recently William Glaser has examined the politics of physician fee negotiations (1978) and the politics of federal-state relations in health-systems management (1979). These studies tend to view health-policy problems as conflicts among established and powerful groups.

Through an eclectic use of research materials, with heavy reliance on elite interviews, they try to explain why one group wins or predict which group will win. Marmor and associates' work has postulated a theoretical framework (based on an analysis of the resources of the competing groups). Glaser's work is more inductive; he establishes a basic description of a particular conflict in a large number of countries (usually around 8 or 10), from which he derives generalizations about the conditions that favor various groups. Both types of studies are able to generalize about the impact of resource distribution or administrative arrangements on the relative power of competing groups. And, as Glaser points out (1978, pp. 243-245), cross-national studies give an excellent opportunity to discover some of the unanticipated consequences of policies and programs that policymakers might be contemplating.

Formats for Presenting Lessons

Comparative health-policy research is usually conducted by academics and presented in academic formats. But the typical academic report is unlikely to be used by policymakers. Books are too long, and academic journal articles, with their literature reviews, methodological sections, and lengthy analysis of data, are absolutely unsuited to the information needs of policymakers. Academic reports must be almost translated, or at least converted, into other formats. Several considerations should guide these translations.

The writer should have in mind a specific audience. The audience should be those who will not only find the lessons useful but who are in an institutional position to implement the lessons. Thus, for example, if the results provide strategic lessons on how to pass cost-control legislation, the writing should be aimed at legislators and lobbyists. By thinking about the formal authority and informal political resources of the audience, the writer can present lessons that are more useful to policymakers.

The results of lesson-drawing research should be packaged for the use of busy, action-oriented people who do not share the scholar's leisurely attitude toward reading. It goes without saying that the writing should be brief. More important, the organization must be very different from that of scholarly writing. Many devices of academic writing are inappropriate in policy writing—introductions that set the context of the problem, reviews of previous scholarly work, detailed presentations of data, flowing transition sentences, and gradual, suspense-building approaches to the conclusion. If lesson-drawing research is to reach the people who can act on it, the conclusions must come first. If the policymaker reads nothing but the first sentence, he or she should at least know the main lesson before he is distracted by the next item of business. Conclusions and recommendations should even be visually distinguishable from the supporting evidence and contextual discussions; underlining, headings, different typefaces are all devices that can be used.

If scholars setting out to do comparative health-policy research considered the potential audience and imagined the final packaging of their research in these ways, chances are good that the research they did would be designed to produce more usable lessons. Perhaps if every researcher concluded his or her study with an option memorandum to a responsible official in health policy, the field would move a long way in the direction of constructive lesson drawing.

References

Adams, James L. 1974. *Conceptual Blockbusting.* San Francisco: Freeman.

Alford, Robert. 1975. *Health Care Politics*. Chicago: University of Chicago Press.

Bryant, John. 1969. *Health and the Developing World*. Ithaca: Cornell University Press. Cited in Elling 1980, p. 47.

Elling, Ray. 1980. *Cross-National Studies of Health Systems*. New Brunswick: Transaction Books.

Field, Mark. 1976. "The Need for Cross-National Studies in Health Services," in *Cross National Sociomedical Research: Concepts, Methods, Practice*, M. Pflanz and E. Schach, eds. Stuttgart: Thieme, pp. 3-11.

Glaser, William. 1979. "Federalism in Canada and West Germany, Lessons for the United States," unpublished manuscript, Center for the Social Sciences, Columbia University, New York.

_____. 1978. *Health Insurance Bargaining: Foreign Lessons for Americans*. New York: Wiley.

_____. 1977. "The Process of Cross-national Survey Research," in *Cross-national Comparative Survey Research*, L.A. Azalai and R. Petrella, eds. New York: Pergamon Press, pp. 403-435.

Harris, Richard. 1966. *A Sacred Trust*. New York: New American Library.

Jonsson, Egon, and Neuhauser, Duncan. 1975 "Hospital Staffing Ratios in the United States and Sweden," *Inquiry* 12:128-137.

Kohn, Robert, and Kerr, L. White. 1976. *Health Care an International Study: Report of the WHO International Collaborative Study of Medical Care Utilization*. New York: Oxford University Press.

Lembcke, Paul. 1959. "Hospital Efficiency: A Lesson From Sweden," *Hospitals* 33:34-38 and 92.

Lubove, Roy. 1968. *The Struggle for Social Security*. Cambridge, Mass.: Harvard University Press.

Marmor, Theodore, Bridges, Amy, and Bickart, Tony. 1980. "American Health Planning and the Lessons of Comparative Policy Analysis," *Journal of Health Politics, Policy and Law* 5.

Marmor, Theodore, and Thomas, David. 1972. "Doctors, Politics and Pay Disputes," *British Journal of Political Science* 2:421-442.

Marmor, Theordore, and Thomas, David. 1971. "The Politics of Paying Physicians: The Determinants of Government Payment Programs in England, Sweden and the United States," *International Journal of Health Services* 1:71-78.

Marmor, Theodore, Wittman, Donald, and Heagy, Thomas. 1976. "The Politics of Medical Inflation," *Journal of Health Politics, Policy and Law* 1:69-84.

Myers, George. 1976. "Mortality Statistics," in *Cross-national Sociomedical Research*, M. Pflanz and E. Schach, eds. Stuttgart: Thieme, pp. 82-93.

Przeworski, Adam, and Teune, Henry. 1970. *The Logic of Comparative Social Inquiry*. New York: Wiley.

Roemer, Milton. 1977. *Comparing National Health Policies*. New York: Marcel Dekker.

Stark, Evan. 1977. "The Epidemic as a Social Event," *International Journal of Health Sciences* 7:681-705.

Stone, Deborah. 1979. "Health Care Cost Containment in the Federal Republic of Germany," *Journal of Health Politics, Policy and Law* 4:176-199.

U.S. Government Accounting Office. 1980. *FDA Drug Approval—A Lengthy Process that Delays the Availability of Important New Drugs.*

12 Planning versus Prevention: Lessons from the USSR

Raisa B. Deber

The ideological skeletons may hang in separate cupboards, but the same political wind rattles both sets of bones. —R. Pinker, *Social Theory and Social Policy*

As the share of national income consumed by the health-care sector rises, there has been an increasing perception of a "crisis" in medical care.[1] This crisis has been variously defined as: "excessive costs," "inadequate accessibility," or "poor value for money"; perceived causes have included inadequate competition among providers, the inefficiency of a nonmarket sector of the economy, or the insatiable nature of human demands for medical services. The problem of how to provide "needed" services as economically, equitably, and efficiently as possible has arisen cross-nationally; no existing health-care system appears to have "solved" the problem of defining and providing an "appropriate" level of services. In the United States, however, the problem has become more acute as third-party payers (particularly governments) have eliminated most financial constraints on the growth of the health-care sector.[2] American health-status indicators are no better than those of nations spending far less proportionally for health care. Fears that instituting national health insurance, without fundamental reforms in the organization of the health-care system, would further increase costs without corresponding benefits, have led to a search for the "quick fix." Among the potential panaceas suggested are planning and prevention.

Why Planning?

Both planning and prevention have an underlying rationale of increasing the efficiency with which services are provided. Planning has been defined by Blum as "having the purposes of:

Specifying what is wanted.

Attaining what is wanted by means of designing plans and strategies for accomplishment.

Measuring the degree of success in attaining what was desired."[3]

Planning can be analyzed in many ways. Some authors view planning as

149

a rational method of matching resources to needs, while avoiding waste and duplication. "The unexamined underlying premise of this view of health planning is that voluntary cooperation among providers, based on reliable information furnished by a disinterested agency, would suffice to meet the public interest."[4] Planning has been justified by others as providing a regulatory mechanism that can compensate for the inability of market economics, under prevailing conditions of consumer ignorance and third-party payment, to lead to optimal results in the health-care field. Others have focused on the impact of the planning exercise—as a change in the rules of the game—upon the distribution of power. They note that any planning exercise, by stressing access to data and command over analytic techniques, may shift power from field practitioners to central agencies such as regulatory bodies or central administration. Still others have focused on the mechanics of health planning. For example, Klarman stressed the structure of the health-planning organizations, the procedures they follow, and the functions they are intended to perform.[5]

One crucial distinction in analyzing the potential impact of planning on health programs is whether planning is seen as only providing *information* about needs and resources; as setting *desired* levels of service, methods of organization, or types of programs; as being a *guide* to resource allocation; or as being a rational *plan* for action. Although "measuring the degree of success in attaining what was desired" implies a necessity for monitoring outcomes, this monitoring becomes crucial if feedback mechanisms are to be employed to alter actions and/or planning targets. Accordingly, much of the attention of health planners has been devoted to the development of data systems and health indicators to facilitate such monitoring.[6]

A considerable literature exists on the informational requirements of a monitoring system, which can be sizeable. Much criticism of recent health-planning legislation and of the PSRO movement has concentrated on the resources required to gather the required data and the extent to which such resource utilization is cost effective. Some critics have also recognized that there is considerable variation in the ease with which outcomes can be measured and that a danger exists of skewing one's efforts toward what can be measured. Intangibles are not always inconsequentials. This concern has been pervasive in the quality-of-care literature, for example, where the early realization that health outcomes—purportedly the subject of concern—were ambiguously related to health inputs, inconveniently far removed from those inputs in time (particularly when speaking of chronic diseases), and inherently difficult to measure has led to a concentration on measuring inputs (for example, numbers of doctors, hospitals, utilization statistics) or process (for example, medical audit) as a more manageable, but questionable, substitute.[7] Program evaluation, as a field, is also aware of the dangers of evaluating only those outcomes that are easily measured, at the risk of ignoring the most important goals of an organization or program. A related danger is the skewing of programs toward outcomes that can be evaluated in the short run, at the possible expense of more crucial, but long-term, outcomes.

This skewing effect becomes the object of concern, as limited resources may preclude spending on both what can be measured and what is important but ill defined. In the case of public goods such as public health, which are classic examples of goods that are difficult to define and measure, the question of where to direct one's efforts in the absence of market cues becomes even more acute.

Prevention

An alternative to planning the number and distribution of resources needed to care for illness is to eliminate the causes of disease. The imagery of infectious disease has been seductive. Clearly, polio was treated far more effectively through eliminating the disease—that is, immunization—than through planning regional networks of respirators. By analogy, policymakers have hoped that other diseases could also be eliminated, removing the need for expensive treatment facilities. This approach was popularized by the Lalonde Report in Canada,[8] and has been accompanied by calls for antistress, diet modification, antismoking, proexercise, antialcohol, and other forms of lifestyle alteration, as well as by the environmental and occupational health movements.

Although its vision of a disease-free life through sensible living has been overstated, prevention does hold out some slender hopes of reducing at least some short-term demands on the health-care system.[9]

Prevention programs have commonly been categorized as follows:

1. Primary prevention, consisting of health promotion, and specific protection
2. Secondary prevention, consisting of early diagnosis and prompt treatment, and disability limitation
3. Tertiary prevention, or rehabilitation.[10]

In order to operationalize and evaluate a preventive program, one must confront an important philosophical problem: What is the meaning of a nonevent?

Evaluation of *any* program would in theory involve looking at how many people were serviced by it, and how well the program met their needs. In collecting the relevant data, one must then ascertain how separable the outcome is from the process of monitoring it. In the case of health-related data, that question involves several aspects.

1. What is the time lag until the onset of disease? For some conditions, the

time lag between exposure and onset may be 20 years or more. Thus current data reflect ancient practices; conversely, it may not be possible to evaluate actions taken now until far in the future. Such time lags present obvious problems in evaluating the short-term effectiveness of a program.

2. How clear cut is the event? When, for example, does a cavity need to be filled? What level of blood pressure requires treatment for hypertension? To the extent that ambiguity exists about when a condition needs to be treated, statistics about need are susceptible to variation across observers.

3. How easily detected is the event? Is the condition one for which people will seek out treatment or is outreach a factor? To the extent that the condition is asymptomatic (for example, hypertension), then prevalence and incidence rates will depend on the extent of casefinding.

To the extent that providers may have incentives to find more, perhaps borderline, cases, there may be a necessity for incorporating an independent monitoring source. To the extent that disease statistics are susceptible to distortion through the reporting process, it becomes difficult to know how effective a program has been.

In the case of preventive programs, as already mentioned, the situation is complicated by the fact that one is inherently dealing with nonevents. If one does not observe an event—for example, if fewer people use the services of a clinic—there are three possibilities: The potential patients were served by another clinic; a smaller number of people needed the services of the clinic; or there were a number of people who needed but did not receive medical services. In the first case, the total number of services received within the community would be unchanged, and the macro planning implications would involve, at most, a reallocation of resources. On the micro level the program being investigated should be considered unsuccessful, as demonstrated in unambiguous market terms (the customers went elsewhere). In the second case, there has been a successful example of prevention, which led to a decreased need for curative services. In the third case, needs have not been met, and there is an increased need for curative resources, and possibly for increases in outreach programs. Simple observation of the number of people served by the clinic does not enable one to distinguish among these possibilities.

For such programs, it is operationally impossible to distinguish (particularly on the basis of data internal to the program) between success and failure.

Such dilemmas are not unique to health policy. In the field of law enforcement, crime statistics are notoriously susceptible to recording practices, and the eagerness with which lawbreakers are sought out ("outreach programs," of sorts). A small number of traffic tickets may indicate a law-abiding citizenry, a low priority placed on traffic laws by the police force, a ticket fixer in the department, or traffic police sleeping on the job. Improving law enforcement may therefore lead to an increase in the number of tickets. Similarly, the success or failure rates of students may indicate more about the grading practices of teachers than about the amount of education that has occurred. The high degree of discretion in recording events—the interaction between observer and observed—ensures that nonevents do not have an easily interpreted meaning.

What then occurs when one attempts to plan and monitor a program of prevention? To the extent that genuine prevention would imply the nonoccurrence of events, such programs would be extremely difficult to monitor. To the extent that a health-planning system required such monitoring, it would be predicted that such programs would be poorly received by funding and administrative personnel in the competition for scarce resources. The desire to monitor outcomes would instead favor programs whose outputs were easily defined and measured. In the area of prevention, this theory would predict that prevention would become defined in terms of screening, testing, or treating identifiable units, such that goals could be set and met.

To explore this theory, an investigation was made of the health-care system of the USSR, a society whose health system is explicitly centered around central planning and around prevention.

The USSR

"What are the Basic Principles of the Soviet Health System? These can be summed up as follows: socialised medicine under state control; free and accessible health services; disease prevention, and a democratic approach to health prevention."[11]

The Soviets use the term "public health" to refer to the entire network of health-care services, including hospitals, spas, research institutes and laboratories, child-care centers, and sanatoria as well as traditional public-health activities. The educational system for medical workers is also under the control of the USSR Ministry of Public Health. To the outside observer, a number of features of the Soviet health-care system are striking, including: the regional organization of health-care services, with well-organized referral networks, and a separation of primary, secondary, and tertiary care; the large number of physicians involved in primary care; the wide and systematic provision of continuing education; the high proportion of women as doctors; the low salaries paid to most physicians; the absence of official fee-for-service medicine; the emphasis on planning; and the very high ratios of doctors and beds per capita. The health-care system of the USSR has been summarized in a number of recent studies.[12]

Within the USSR, the health sector is classified as a "nonproductive" part of the economy. It is justified both on humanitarian grounds and on the realization that the productive sectors rely on a healthy workforce. Resources have been allocated accordingly. For example, health services for industrial workers had historical priority over health services for the rest of the population. Heavy emphasis was also placed on the conquest of infectious disease—as Lenin said, "Either socialism will defeat the louse, or the louse will defeat socialism."[13] Given the scarcity of health resources at the time of the Russian revolution, the government policies of enlarging and redistributing the numbers and types of resources has led to dramatic improvements in health status. The Soviet Union now has mortality rates similar to those in Canada and the United States. Nonetheless, the USSR must still cope with infectious diseases (for example, tuberculosis) that are no longer a major factor in western health systems.[14]

Planning in the USSR

The health-care system, like the rest of the Soviet economy, is centrally planned, and centrally directed. As such, it is controlled by "goals" (indicators). Overall plan goals are set by the central Soviet planning authority (Gosplan), based on figures provided by local authorities. In an elaborate mechanism, plans are sent up and down the chain of command. Ultimately, factories will be given production quotas; doctors will have plan targets for the number of patient visits, house calls, and X-rays; research workers will have plan targets for the number of compounds they should synthesize. These targets are customarily derived "from the achieved level," that is, incrementally.[15] Plan targets are thus difficult to alter, particularly given the nature of relationships with suppliers in a planned economy. There is also strong incentive to *achieve* plan targets. Bonuses are dependent on plan fulfillment; managers may find their jobs in jeopardy if plan targets have not been met.

Soviet health planning is complex and sophisticated. Soviet authorities have defined the discipline as dealing, in a scientific manner, with

1. Methods and organization of work
2. Lowering morbidity and improving public-health status
3. Standards for medical services to the public (including bed and doctor ratios)
4. Plans for development of public-health networks and location of health institutions
5. Manpower
6. Medical scientific research
7. The material and technical base of public-health and scientific medical institutions

It therefore encompasses medical education, medical research, appropriate staffing ratios, "work norms" for staff members, and is allied to public-health economics, the role of public health in the development of the national economy, an economic evaluation of forms and methods of providing medical services to the public, the economics of medical institutions (especially hospitals), and public-health financing. The health indicators must be meshed with other aspects of the national health plan, including net expenditures, the operational requirements for wages, number of employees, fuel and energy, various industrial and agricultural products, and needs for building materials, machines and workers, and capital funds.[16]

The planning authorities of the All-Union (national) Ministry of Health have devoted considerable attention to "scientific organization and planning" of health services. For example, time-motion types of studies have been conducted for medical practitioners, and the amount of time that "should" be spent with a patient has been calculated. Demands have been computed, often through surveys of morbidity or other examinations of utilization patterns. Some of these studies have tried to capture "hidden" morbidity for which treatment was not sought, although these studies were flawed methodologically. As a result of such studies, the Ministry of Health has computations for how many patients will require services of each type, what medical specialists/personnel are required (or even preferred) to perform such services, and how many of such services they can perform in a given time period. From such data, it is a simple mathematical calculation to determine the numbers and deployment of resources necessary to meet the health needs of the community.

Given these calculations and norms, plus demographic data for the local catchment area, the public-health plan is able to specify quite closely what utilization should be for each health unit by category of service. Although the results can be criticized for the underlying specialty-based, curative assumptions,[17] they are excellent examples of planning at its most grandiose.

The requirements for monitoring in the Soviet system are cumbersome. In the case of health, the informational demands result in a good deal of physicians's time being taken up with record keeping and paperwork.[18]

One weakness in a planned system is a slugishness in responding to innovation. There are high transaction costs associated with change; and it is therefore difficult to get an adaptive and creative response.[19] Most writers on the Soviet system have documented a massive resistance to change.

What, then, are the implications of the planning system for preventive programs?

Prevention

To evaluate prevention in the USSR, several points should be noticed. First, sanitary and epidemiological services have long been separated from curative medicine. Sanitation and hygiene (public health) doctors are educated in a separate stream.[20] In 1973 only 45,000 of 766,700 physicians in the USSR were specialists in public health and epidemiology.[21] Administratively, curative medicine is delivered through a network of ambulatory clinics and a separate network of referral hospitals, both of which are administered and operated by local governments. Another network of clinics and hospitals are located, administered, and operated by industrial firms for the treatment of their workers. Traditional public health is conducted by a network of over 5000 "sanepids" (sanitational and epidemiological stations) that have responsibility for eradication and curtailment of infectious diseases, for occupational health, and some responsibilities for child health, nutrition, and environmental health and sanitation. On paper, they have impressive authority, including the right to shut down a workplace or destroy defective products. However, much occupational health is conducted by the curative network since hospitals and primary-care physicians are located within many workplaces and will provide all medical care (not just for job-related disorders) to workers and often to workers' families. The regional health-care institutions (district clinics and so on) are, in many cases, only for those without access to health care through their workplace.

Second, as in the West, prevention and public health have less prestige than does curative medicine. The preeminence of the hospital (which has even at times received responsibility for delivery of primary care and preventive services) has implied a lower priority for preventive services. For example, the chief doctor of the district hospital is in charge of all medical care for his district (including some responsibility for allocating budgets and planned targets among the medical organizations). The chief epidemiological doctor is his deputy. Curative hospital-based services are thus recognized as the controlling sector of medicine. Conclusions about the Soviet health-care system must therefore be modified by the high emphasis that they have placed on traditional curative medicine and on specialists.[22]

A major method by which the Soviets dispense preventive care is through "dispensarization" (surveillance with medical-record linkage). This involves regular check-ups and prophylactic treatment for designated chronic diseases of all people in the specified categories and client groups. These categories include disabled war veterans, hypertensives, those with gastrointenstinal ailments, diabetes, cancer, tuberculosis, as well as those referred by outpatient clinics, and "high-risk" elements of the healthy population such as children, adolescents, students, pregnant women, and the majority of industrial, office, and agricultural workers. "Definite intervals in the administration of medical and prophylactic treatment have been established for each group.[23] A newspaper article, noticing the higher mortality and morbidity rates among men, suggested that "men of all ages—and especially older men—should be given a place of high priority (along with women who work in unfavorable conditions) in receiving health care."[24]

Sizeable resources have been devoted to dispensarization and other forms of screening. "The Ministry of Health network of dispensaries exceeded 3,700 in 1971, or which 1,373 were for tuberculosis, 772 for venereal and dermatological diseases, 269 for cancer and 247 for psychiatry and neurology. Over 9.5 million adults and adolescents attended dispensaries in urban areas in 1965 (1.12 mn for hypertension, 0.71 mn for rheumatism and 0.62 for stomach and duodenal ulcers). Screenings and periodic health checks in that year included 10.48 million workers in industrial enterprises, 5.2 million workers in food, sanitation, child care and health care institutions, 2.81 million apprentices and students and 22.20 million schoolchildren, the total number in 1971 was 101 million."[25] Government policies were set that all non-TB patients should have a chest X-ray every two years and that all women over age twenty-five be screened for cancer every six months.[26]

"In 1966, over 70 percent of the population aged 30 and over were given routine medical examinations for the detection of malignant growths. Of every thousand people examined nine were registered as having precancer conditions such as polyposis of the gastrointestinal tract, erosion of the uterine cervix, pathology of the mammary glands, and dermal neoplasms."[27] High priority was given in the 5-year plan of 1970 to extending and improving the dispensary method of service to the population.[28] By 1974 the number of people under dispensary observation had increased by 2.1 million over the previous year, to 32.5 million. Ryan noted that "although Soviet bureaucrats and clinicians alike appear to be convinced that results justify the resources required, so far as the author is aware, conventional wisdom in this matter has not been subjected to fundamental appraisal."[29]

It should be noted that the dispensaries are specialized by disease type. Although this may be justified in terms of treatment, (TB dispensaries, for example, contain operating facilities), when the outreach function is added, it may involve many different groups, each checking the same patient for their particular disease.

It has been recognized that screening for low-prevalence diseases requires an inordinate amount of input and is rarely cost effective.[30] To the extent that follow-up measures resulting (prescribed) from a positive test are detrimental to health, the cumulative effect of screening to the health of a community may be negative—the effects on the high proportion of false positives outweighing the benefits to those with the disease. From the standpoint of achieving goals, however, this strategy has the advantages of setting clear, countable goals that can be increased for subsequent planning periods. If all women are screened for breast cancer every six months, a new goal can add screening for cervical cancer, or Herpes virus, or diabetes. Age groups to be screened can be expanded, screening intervals shortened, false positives investigated more thoroughly, or diagnostic tests added. Prevention can become a fertile source of increased needs and justify an increased flow of resources into the health sector.

At least in the published work (in English) of Soviet health planners (as well as in their talks with me), there was little sensitivity to problems of screening and little attention to the nature of demand. For example, Zhuk looked forward to the day when the whole population would come under dispensary observation, and health planners would therefore have good statistics on morbidity based on population surveys.[31] His discussion, which was fairly uncritical of screening, concentrated on the problems of underutilization of services. The hypothesis of physician-generated demand and the differentiation between demand and need was not evident. When decreases in length of stay were discussed by Soviet health planners, it was with a view toward the number of additional patients who could be treated, and the effective number of "new beds" created; closing beds was discussed only in conjunction with merging too-small facilities to create larger units. The belief that the way to improved health care was to increase the number of visits, the time per visit, or the quality of doctors (through increased education, for example) was pervasive.

Accordingly, public-health goals are often set in terms of increasing countable numbers. The *Current Digest of the Soviet Press* contains many examples from the Soviet press. "The USSR Council of Ministers has adopted a resolution On Measures for the Further Improvement of Opthalmological Services to the Public. . . . The resolution provides for . . . further developing the network of departments, offices and centers that provide emergency opthalmological treatments at hospitals and polyclinics. . . [and] for extensive preventive examinations of the public for the purpose of early detection of eye diseases."[32] Other decrees call for increasing the number of medical examinations to be given to children, for the elderly, increasing numbers of hospital beds, and so on.

A similar urge to increase the utilization of services can be seen in a medical campaign against self-treatment. In one article, the concerns extended beyond discouraging the use of quack medicines. The chairman of the board of the All-Union Scientific Society of Therapists included warnings that "much harm can be caused by uncontrolled jogging, plunging into ice holes to cure the body . . . and excessive use of saunas." The authors continue, "We feel that the ineffectiveness of some types of therapy, the resistance some microbes develop to medicines, the increasing frequency of allergic reactions and instances in which acute diseases become chronic are in large measure a consequence of treatment that is not supervised by physicians. . . . One of the main tasks of medical education is to prevent erroneous actions on the part of the patient or those around him." They concluded, "All this brings to light the main flaw in our efforts at general medical education: In populuar articles, books, lectures and discussions we still do a poor job of teaching the population to seek prompt medical assistance."[33]

This tendency to define health care, including prevention, in terms that are countable and increasable can be seen in the Soviet antismoking programs. Although the antismoking programs in the USSR include a number of components such as educational programs and selective bans on smoking, they rely quite heavily on screening and one-on-one medical treatment by a specialist physician.[34] What they do not include, however, is direct action against cigarettes—bans on their sale. The antialcohol programs similarly include labor-intensive voluntary-treatment programs for alcoholics—a minimum of 45 days inpatient treatment (including drug treatment and psychotherapy), followed up by to six months of "labor therapy," when the alcoholic is living at the clinic and working at an attached factory. These patients are then "registered" and followed up for five years; recidivists may have to repeat the whole process. Another network of guarded clinics (with attached factories) under the Ministery of Internal Affairs treats patients who have been sentenced to treatment by a court. Five-year cure rates were reported to be about one third (60 percent for voluntary patients.)[35]

On the face of it, it appears irrational that one hand of the Soviet government is trying to eliminate the consumption of tobacco products while the other hand is sponsoring research on improving yields of tobacco,[36] in designing more attractive cigarette packages, and in distributing them in the stores. Similarly, one hand of the government of the USSR campaigns against alcoholism while the other continues to manufacture high-alcohol, low-quality fortified wine.[37] It is necessary to recognize that both hands are connected to planning agencies and have a need to meet plan goals. Thus a decrease in the number of cigarettes consumed would threaten directly the ability of the relevant departments to meet their sales quotas. A shift from sweet to dry wine would imperil city budgets, which collect taxes on the basis of alcohol content; threaten the ability of wine manufacturers to meet their quotas for sweet wines, reverberate to the needs of sugar manufacturers (who dispose of some of their sales to the winemakers), of bottle manufacturers, and the like. Any change not only threatens a network of stable relationships, it jeopardizes the ability to meet plan targets. Although true prevention would have a difficult-to-measure impact on public-health goals, it would detectably threaten the ability of other segments of the economy to achieve plan fulfillment.

On the other hand, medical treatment of smokers or drinkers can be evaluated in terms of how many smokers or drinkers are being serviced. Both programs have excellent potential for requiring trained specialists to extend the programs to all smokers or drinkers; neither demand changes in the activities of other sectors of the economy.

It is also clear that public-health authorities would prefer concrete, meetable goals (for example, number of inspections performed) to fuzzier goals over whose fulfillment they would have less control (for example, concentration of a particular pollutant that might have been generated in a different jurisdiction.)

What then can one note about Soviet health activities? One would predict that action against pollution would be less popular than screening the victims of pollution. Indeed, scholars have concluded that the Soviet record on pollution appears to be as bad as that of most capitalist countries. The Soviets have had difficulty in implementing health-related goals when these conflict with increased production. Housing and pollution control are the responsibilities of local authorities, and conflict with the interests of large industrial enterprises, which are not under the direct control of local authorities. Taubman found industrialization was sacred over almost everything else, with a consequent disregard for pollution, occupational health, sanitation, and housing.[38]

One could also predict that the pseudo-reality of meeting planning targets would take precedence over the more elusive true requirements of a situation. As one example, because departments kept data only on *total* wine sold, progress could be shown in the campaign to combat drunkenness by encouraging drinkers to shift from vodka to wine, whether or not alcoholism, or even alcohol consumption, had been reduced. As a Soviet reporter noted, this progress was illusory; most of the increased wine consumption was of low-quality fortified wines, and crimes related to drunkenness appeared to have increased. The reporter concluded, "Now the time has come to . . . evaluate the true merits of the departmental indices, which at first glance seem effective but ultimately cause enormous social losses."[39]

Implications

It has been concluded that a monitored bureau must "consume more and more of its resources to satisfy the demands of the monitors for information . . . and devote ever more resources to figuring out ways of evading or counteracting the monitor's additional regulations."[40] "The essential point . . . is that in most instances *the center does not know* just what it is that needs doing, in disaggregated detail, while the management in its situation *cannot* know what it is that society needs unless the centre informs it." Despite all talk of reform and direct links, the fact remains that in a basically nonmarket model, the center must discover what needs doing, and the center *cannot* do this in microdetail. At the same time the center pursues its own priorities, including growth. To encourage growth it sets objectives, goals, and rewards their attainment. These targets are expressed in aggregate terms, inevitably. The attempt by management to obey plan instructions, which gives rise to many distortions, is not evidence of lack of common interest; if anything it is the reverse. The trouble lies in the near impossibility of drafting microeconomic instructions in such a way that even the most well-meaning manager will not be misled.[41]

If one is to run a monitoring system, it is necesary to set goals. If one is to succeed in a system that is being monitored, it is necessary to meet the goals that have been set. It would be irrational for practitioners to design a program with goals that would be difficult to meet. From this it can be inferred that the nature of the goals will affect the activities of the participants in the system. For example, if it is desired to curb child abuse, one form of goal setting would be a planned decrease in the number of child-abuse cases that are treated. To the extent that the diagnosis of child abuse is not unambiguous, the easiest way to meet this goal would be to misclassify child-abuse cases (for example, as accidents). Statistics about alcoholism, suicide, drug abuse, venereal disease, and mental illness would be similarly susceptible to reporting error. To the extent that central authorities are alert to this possibility, they may either superimpose another monitoring system to check the validity of the statistics gathered, or choose to set goals where there is less of an incentive to understate events. "Low-ball" sorts of goals may be equally unattractive from a funding standpoint since it is politically vulnerable, and psychologically unattractive, to pay someone for not doing something (that is, not treating cases of child abuse.)[42]

An alternative, more attractive strategy is to set goals whose achievement can be measured in terms of doing more, not less. Screening programs are desirable in these terms. An expanded program against breast cancer then could be measured in the numbers of women who have received mammograms, been taught breast self-examination, received a pamphlet, and so on, rather than by decreases in mortality rates from breast cancer (statistics that would, at any rate, take many years to show an impact.)

The potential must not be forgotten that an attempt to increase rationality, through a reliance on health planning, may paradoxically make health-care services *less* efficient if a concentration on monitorable, short-term outcomes leads to an abandonment of programs that may have significant long-range impacts but whose effects are difficult to measure in the short term.

Notes

1. John H. Knowles, ed., *Doing Better and Feeling Worse: Health in the United States* (New York: Norton, 1977).

2. D.P. Rice, and D. Wilson, "The American Medical Economy: Problems and Perspectives," *Journal of Health Politics, Policy and Law* 1(2) (Summer 1976):151-172.

3. Henrik L. Blum, *Planning for Health: Development and Application of Social Change Theory* (New York: Human Sciences Press, 1974), p. 111.

4. H. Klarman, "Health Planning: Progress, Prospects and Issues," *Milbank Memorial Fund Quarterly* 56(1) (1978):78-112.

5. Klarman, "Health Planning"; P.N. Reeves, D.F. Bergwall, and N.B. Woodside, *Introduction to Health Planning*, 2nd ed. (Washington, D.C.: Information Resources Press, 1979); David E. Berry, "The Transfer of Planning Theories to Health Planning Practice," *Policy Sciences* 5 (1974):343-361.

6. See, for example, J. Elinson, A. Mooney, and A.E. Siegmann, eds., *Health Goals and Health Indicators: Policy, Planning, and Evaluation* (Boulder, Col.: Westview Press, 1977).

7. R.H. Brook, *Quality of Care Assessment: A Comparison of Five Methods of Peer Review* (U.S. Department of Health, Education, and Welfare, Public Health Service, Health Resources Administration, 1973); C.E. Lewis, "The State of the Art of Quality Assessment—1973," *Medical Care* 12(10) (1974):799-806; R.H. Brook, and F.A. Appel, "Quality-of-care Assessment: Choosing a Method for Peer Review," *New England Journal of Medicine* 288(25) (21 June 1973):1323-1329.

8. M. Lalonde, *A New Perspective on the Health of Canadians: A Working Document* (Ottawa: Department of National Health and Welfare, 1974).

9. J.E. Fielding, "Successes of Prevention," *Milbank Memorial Fund Quarterly* 56(3) (Summer 1979):274-302; Robert W. Morgan, *Prospects for Preventive Medicine: A Catalogue* (Toronto, Ontario: Ontario Economic Council Occasional Paper 2, 1977). It should be recognized, however, that given the expected increase in the proportion of elderly and the accompanying increases in demands on the health-care system, even postponing the demands for care may be expected to increase health-care costs. G.B. Gori and B.J. Richter, "Macroeconomics of Disease Prevention in the United States," *Science* 200 (4346) (1978):1124-1130.

10. Hugh Rodman Leavell and E. Gurney Clark, eds., *Preventive Medicine for the Doctor in his Community: An Epidemiologic Approach*, 3rd ed. (New York: McGraw-Hill 1965), chap. 2.

11. Nikolai Shesternya, *U.S.S.R. Yesterday, Today, Tomorrow. Health Protection* (Moscow: Novosti Press Agency Publishing House, 1976).

12. V.V. Golovteyev, "Complex Long- and Short-term Planning on Health Development in the USSR," pp. 77-80 in N.T.J. Bailey and M. Thompson, *Systems Aspects of Health Planning*, Proceedings of the IIASA Conference, Baden, Austria, (August 20-22), 1974, Amsterdam: North-Holland Publishing Company, 1975; M. Kaser, *Health Care in the Soviet Union and Eastern Europe* (London: Croom Helm, 1976); V. Navarro, *Social Security and Medicine in the USSR: A Marxist Critique* (Lexington, Mass.: LexingtonBooks, D.C. Heath, 1977); M. Ryan, *The Organization of Soviet Medical Care* (Oxford: Basil Blackwell and London: Martin Robertson, 1978).

13. Navarro, *Social Security*, pp. 24-25.

14. Kaser, *Health Care in the Soviet Union.*

15. I. Birman, "From the Achieved Level," *Soviet Studies* 30(2) (1978): 153-172; A. Nove, *The Soviet Economic System* (London: George Allen and Unwin Ltd., 1977).

16. A.P. Zhuk, *Public Health Planning in the U.S.S.R.,* translated from the Russian language and reproduced in limited quantities by the Geographic Health Studies Program of the John E. Fogarty International Center for Advanced

Study in the Health Sciences, USDHEW, Public Health Service, DHEW Publication No. 76-999, 1976.

17. Navarro, *Social Security*.

18. The figure of 60 percent is given by Slinin. S. Slinin, "Write or Treat? Once Again About the Physician's Work Time," *Izvestia*, 11 February 1978, p. 2, from *Current Digest of the Soviet Press (CDSP)* vol. 30 (no. 6) (8 March 1978).

19. Richard R. Nelson, *The Moon and The Ghetto: An Essay on Public Policy Analysis* (New York: Norton, 1977).

20. In 1938 medical studies were divided into three main branches: general medicine (therapy and industrial preventive medicine), maternity and child care, and sanitation and hygiene (public health). Navarro, *Social Security*, p. 47.

21. Kaser, *Health Care in the Soviet Union*, p. 83.

22. Navarro, *Social Security*; Ryan, *Organization of Soviet Medical Care*.

23. Shesternya, *U.S.S.R.*, p. 25.

24. B. Urlanis, "Once Again Cherish the Men!" *Literaturnaya gazeta*, 7 June 1978. In *CDSP*, 30(24) (12 July 1978):16.

25. Kaser, *Health Care in the Soviet Union*, pp. 59-60.

26. *Medical Care in the USSR: Report of the U.S. Delegation on Health Care Services and Planning*, 16 May-3 June 1970. U.S. Department of Health, Education and Welfare, Public Health Service/National Institutes of Health. DHEW Publication No. NIH 72-60, 1972.

27. Zhuk, *Public Health Planning*, p. 46.

28. USSR CPSU Central Committee and the USSR Council of Ministers, "Resolution on Improving Health Care," *Pravda* and *Izvestia*, 15 October 1977, in *CDSP* 29(41) (9 November 1977):16-18.

29. Ryan, *Organization of Soviet Medical Care*, p. 134.

30. Cf. K.S. Bay, D. Flathman, and L. Nestman, "The Worth of a Screening Program: An Application of a Statistical Decision Model for the Benefit Evaluation of Screening Projects," *American Journal of Public Health* 66(2) (February 1976):145-150; Anne-Marie Foltz, and Jennifer L. Kelsey, "The Annual Pap Test: A Dubious Policy Success," *Milbank Memorial Fund Quarterly* 56(4) (1978):426-457; David Eddy, *Screening for Cancer: Theory, Analysis and Design,"* 1978.

31. Zhuk, *Public Health Planning*, p. 107.

32. *Izvestia*, 25 April 1978, in *CDSP* 30(17) (24 May 1978):19.

33. F. Komarov, and N. Elshtein, "Self-Treatment? No!" *Pravda*, 27 September 1977. In *CDSP* 29(39) (26 October 1977):22-23.

34. Raisa E. Deber, "Anti-Smoking Programmes in the U.S.S.R," *Canadian Journal of Public Health*, in press.

35. Babayon, personal interview, 1978.

36. I. Lukin, "In Neutral Gear," *Pravda*, 26 August 1977, in *CDSP* 29(34) (21 September 1977):20.

37. Vil Dorofeyev, *Literaturnaya gazeta*, 22 February 1978, in *CDSP* 30 (8) (22 March 1978):11-12.

38. Nove, *The Soviet Economic System*, p. 76; Marshall I. Goldman, *The Spoils of Progress: Environmental Pollution in the Soviet Union* (Cambridge, Mass.: MIT Press, 1972); W. Taubman, *Governing Soviet Cities: Bureaucratic Politics and Urban Development in the U.S.S.R.* (New York: Praeger Publishers, 1973).

39. Dorofeyev, *Literaturnaya gazeta*. Counterproductive effects of planning indicators are, of course, not restricted to the USSR. U.S. efforts to curb air and water pollution have been plagued by "successess" that meet targets for reduction of particular pollutants while releasing large quantities of new, often more harmful substances that were not included in the original legislation. Optimism that the problem will be solved once the "right" indicators are devised is becoming less pronounced as the number of possible chemical compounds that could be created is realized.

40. Anthony Downs, *Inside Bureaucracy* (Boston: Little, Brown, 1967).

41. Nove, *The Soviet Economic System*, p. 74.

42. Another example is the difficulty in accepting the principle of capitation payments; newspapers have a tendency to discover such scandals as an HMO where doctors were actually paid a fee for patients they had not seen during the month (see *Toronto Star*, 8 April 1980).

13 Health Care and Political Values

Sondra Z. Koff

While culture has long been a central concern to anthropologists and sociologists, it is only in the past two decades that political scientists have endeavored systematically to study its impact on political life. Particularly in the subfield of comparative politics, political culture has been an important tool of analysis, even though critical attacks have been launched against it. For the most part, these attacks have charged that several properties of the concept create difficulties, especially in the area of measurement. Recognizing its limitations, this chapter will demonstrate how the political-culture approach can aid students of comparative health care in describing and explaining similarities and differences in health-care policy and delivery systems among and within nations.

Various notions of the concept of political culture have been set forth in the literature. For this discussion it is understood as the property of a collectivity that encompasses patterns of orientations of a cognitive, affective, and evaluative nature toward political objects. The objects involve the input and output dimensions of a political system as they relate to health-care policy and the resulting delivery system.[1] Moreover, the distinction between political culture and the general cultural system of a collectivity is not always complete. The two are overlapping and interrelated.

Political culture has an impact on the determination of policy priorities, the policy process as well as the scope and content of government activity. The health-policy sector is closely related to political culture values such as ideology. Political ideologies can either enlarge or restrict the role of government. They help set the policy agenda and determine the boundaries for responses to societal issues. Thereby they restrict the range of options available to a specific population. What might represent appropriate solutions to health-care problems in one society might not be viewed in a similar fashion in another. For example, given the impact of liberalism with its antistatist component on public policy in the United States, issues and demands have been handled in such a way as to restrict the policymaking agenda and to foster solutions to problems within the private sector. The inclination of the United States toward a liberal laissez-faire ideology and the philosophy of individualism help account for the fact that the public provision of health-care services has been less readily accepted than in other nations such as Cuba, the Soviet Union, and England, countries wed to disparate but collectivist-oriented ideologies. In the United States the national government has been reticent to act in the health-care sector on a large scale. Thus the health-care-delivery scene has been primarily characterized by private-sector activity. On the other hand, the liberal ideology in Denmark conditioned by the notion of collective voluntarism has had an altogether different impact. Ito has used ideology to explain the success of the Danish primary health-care system and differences in health-insurance arrangements between Denmark and Sweden.[2]

Structural features of health-care delivery systems as well as fundamental policy principles are related to ideology. One of the strengths of political culture as an analytic tool is that it can be used in conjunction with structural features.[3] One of the major reasons for the lack of success in realizing a transformation of the Italian health-care-delivery system in the post-World War II era is that the forces involved in the policymaking process mirror the divisive cleavages evident in the Italian political culture that serves as a guideline for that process. As a nonconsensual society, the nature of political conflict has made problem solving difficult. Intense divisions rooted in geography, demography, ecology, religion, and social and ideological elements have helped to shape the operation of Italian governmental institutions, political parties, and thus policy outputs.

Republican Italy has been marked by weak coalition governments and political instability. The governmental system has been dominated by an ineffectual parliament containing strong party groups based on ideological foundations that reflect the fragmented political culture. There is an intense competition among the many parties, all of which have a fixed clientele. Parliamentary deadlock and frustration, in part, may be traced to *partitocrazia* (party rule). Moreover, Italian governments have had a tenuous base and *immobilismo* has characterized the political system. It has been difficult to achieve consensus among as well as within the political parties that are marked by extreme internal factionalism. Some commentators have noted that *partitocrazia, correntocrazia* (rule of party factions), and *burocrazia* (the oversized, inefficient public service) serve as major sources of Italy's political problems. Due to the existence of this general situation plus the nature of the rules pertaining to the decision-making process, most legislation emanating from the Italian Parliament in the postwar period is minute in nature and manifests a low degree of interest aggregation. Such is certainly true in terms of health policy.

Di Palma attributes this performance to

> Formal and informal parliamentary rules that leave considerable initiative to minorities, individual representatives, and nonpartisan offices of parliament. The rules constitute significant incentives for majority and opposition groups to put aside divisive and unmanageable issues and to concentrate on ordinary administration and everyday transactions. Thus the parties attain a degree of co-existence in parliament they rarely manage to achieve in the more visible and competitive electoral arena. But the feat is accomplished . . . at the cost of planned legislative action and by leaving out of the legislative agenda the issues that most grievously affect the country . . . .[4]

Thus the achievement of convergence and decisional agreement among the political forces on major issues in general, and health care in particular, has been arduous.

Italy has recently undertaken reform in the hospital sector, and in December of 1978 legislation outlining a complete rennovation of health services was passed. The effectiveness of the former has definitely been hindered by cultural variables. For the most part, political authority and effective decision-making relations are absent as far as the implementation mechanisms are concerned. In the hospital-sector, administration, planning, and governing bodies, being of a collective nature, are composed of representatives of many constituencies including spokesmen for the majority and minority positions within the various levels of local government. Given the fragmented and ideological multiparty system, plus the previously mentioned formation of formal factions within the parties, the structures established by the reform legislation have become highly politicized. Positions on hospital boards are frequently stepping stones to other political roles, and political regularity is more highly valued than the public interest. Also the large size and proliferation identified with these entities have only reenforced existing fragmentation. Often the lack of consensus and the political heterogeneity evident in Italian political institutions pervade various hospital organs as well. The same immobilism and paralysis are often manifested.

It has been difficult to realize hospital reform in Italy because of the nature of the implementation mechanisms. They reflect the clientelism, political divisions, fragmentation, and competing lines of authority evident in the Italian political culture. Also because of these same cultural variables, the legislation related to a complete reform of the health-care system was discussed over a thirty-year period. Although consensus concerning the principles of a global health-care reform has been achieved, it is noteworthy that in order to implement this legislation, more than 70 parliamentary enactments are required in addition to 26 laws for each of the 20 regions, subnational units of Italian government similar to the American state. Given past history, it will definitely be a   long period from legislation to complete implementation, which was unrealistically scheduled for 1 January 1980.

The political-culture approach is useful because it accounts for the participation of certain actors in the policy process and their choice of behavior. The role of particular interest groups, political parties, bureaucracies, and so on, can be identified and considered. These groups have performed different roles in different nations and manifested disparate styles of behavior and various relationships with each other. An examination of these factors can aid students of comparative health-care policy in accounting for disparate content in policy output. The latter must be assessed in the broader context of the constraints of the political culture and the political system.

One of the dimensions of political culture is of a horizontal nature. It deals with individuals' identification with each other. Throughout the world, people have different perceptions of one another that range from mutual trust to hostility. These orientations have an impact on social policy. Titmuss has explained differences in practices concerning blood donation in the United States and England partially on the basis of these attitudes which are also related to the variable of deferential or suspicious attitudes toward authority.[5] In the health-care sector these orientations can affect the patient-provider relationship. For example, statistics concerning malpractice suits illustrate that the British are less litigiose than Americans.[6] In part, this situation results from the deference to authority that permeates the British political culture. A new phenomenon on the Italian health-care scene as of March 1980 is the Court for the Rights of the Sick. Interestingly enough, in about a month's time in Rome over a thousand grievances were filed. This onslaught reflects a fundamental suspicion and alienation evident in the Italian political culture.

An important aspect of political culture is the character of opinion toward governmental output. It has been demonstrated that there are cross-national differences concerning pride in social legislation that includes health policy. For example, Americans and the British are proud of their social legislation, which contrasts with the Italian situation. The Italian citizen, particularly in the South of that nation, does not take pride in the political system or its outputs. In fact, a distrust of public institutions is evident. This orientation is manifested toward health-care institutions as well, and it is especially interesting because the Italians have very extensive social-welfare programs. Recent studies have shown that these negative evaluations are becoming more pronounced. There is a wide gap between popular expectations and perceived governmental performance. In a recent survey 77.6 percent of the sample surveyed assigned great responsibility to the government for the policy area of health assistance, and only 37.0 percent of the sample evaluated governmental action positively.[7] Given this imbalance between popular expectations and perceived policy outcomes, existing alienation is only reinforced.

Within the political culture certain dichotomies may be identified. A central one involves a distinction between the political culture of the elite and that of the masses. Empirical studies undertaken by this author in the United States and Italy[8] have shown that there are major differences in attitudes and beliefs of the decision makers and citizens as they relate to emergency medical services. These differences concerned the need to alter the delivery system, aspects of the system that require attention, barriers to modifications, the citizens' role, planning, and priorities related to the spending of public monies, to cite a few items.

Beliefs concerning governmental output in various sectors of public policy carry important implications. A major goal of any health-care policy is to afford better care to the populace. However, legislation and implementation of programs does not necessarily mean that they will be received in a favorable manner by the public at large if they are not tailored to their desires and attitudes. Empirical studies indicate that the citizenry seems to know what it wants in terms of health-care programs in general. Consequently, it has been argued, "It would behoove planners to find out more about what people want and . . . expect from their medical care system *before* new programs are enacted."[9] It is important to understand consumer and mass orientations before medical systems are designed or operated. Otherwise, they might not be workable. Granted these orientations can be improved upon, diverted, or followed depending on the specific circumstances. However, it is important that they be known prior to undertaking action.[10]

Another division within political cultures is the one that distinguishes those more oriented to modern ways from those who adhere to traditional practices. This dichotomony is reflected in several health-care-delivery systems. For example, in Japan one may note that traditional forms of medicine are still utilized along with more modern ones and that the Japanese health-insurance system is based on traditional social and economic institutions. Moreover, in Cuba, in spite of great efforts by Castro to modernize the health-care system, witch doctors have been integrated within the health services. In Algeria as well traditional practices have conflicted with modern therapy as evidenced by Frantz Fanon's experience with the medicine man.

Moreover, many political cutlures are fragmented on a geographic or regional basis as in the case of Italy where the northern part of the nation that is more economically advanced and wed to a European cultural outlook contrasts with the South that is poor and identified with the Mediterranean culture. This regional division is reflected in the distribution of health-care resources as well as in utilization of services. There is a wide gap between northern and southern Italy as far as the allocation of facilities and personnel is concerned. The same inequalities pertain to many nations such as England and pre-Castro Cuba.

In the case of Italy in the North in some areas there are as many as 12-13 hospital beds per 1000 population, while generally in the less-developed South the ratio is 2.8 per 1000 or even less. Consequently, many Southern Italians travel northward for medical assistance. For example, up to 50 percent of the patients in the region of Lombardy come from the South for treatment involving hospital services. In many northern cities Southerners seeking admission to hospitals form lines during the night. Many carry letters of recommendation from prominent social, political, and religious personages depending on the situation. It is reported that often these letters are important in obtaining hospital admission, which is closely related to clientelism. This migration for medical purposes is due to the deficiency in facilities in southern areas but it also results from the aforementioned lack of trust in the existing structures in these zones. The migratory pattern reflects the basic nature of the parochial political culture that is so characteristic of Southern Italy.

Also related to this attitude of trust, or lack thereof, is the public's perceptions of the status of specific actors—such as providers—within the health-care system. For example, orientations concerning the status of health-care providers are particularly important in terms of staffing a health-care-delivery system. Maldistribution of physicians and a shortage of these providers in many nations exacerbate problems related to the availability of care. Efforts to substitute other types of health-care workers for these providers raise questions concerning health occupational prestige. The latter involves the populace's trust in these workers and the acceptance of nonphysician care as high-quality care as well as the citizens' awareness of differences in training and roles of various health professions, among others. It has been shown that the public is capable of evaluating prestige and hierarchy within the health system. Thus it will "undoubtedly be quick to discern whether attempted changes are real or simply new labels for the old system."[11] Such abilities confirmed in other studies have an impact on the personnel component of a health-care-delivery system.

Another variable inherent in political culture that can be cited in connection with ideology and the study of health services is religion. Moreover, it has been argued that religion is an important value that may be essential for a comprehension of differences in politics and public policy among governmental units.[12] In Israel this variable has had a significant influence on the structure of the health-care-delivery system, medical practice as well as the operation of facilities. A major controversy has involved the autopsy issue, and positions have been taken according to interpretation of religious law. This controversy has created a schism among Israeli physicians that is based on a clerical-anticlerical cleavage. Moreover, dietary customs and other religious practices have had an impact on the cost and size of hospital facilities as well as institutional timetables. In Italy the populace has long been divided along clerical and secular lines, and this cleavage is evident throughout the health-care system, but especially in the emergency-medical-services subsystem. Associations performing onsite service response are frequently identified with the laical or confessional camp. Given the intensity of this religious schism in the political culture, these organizations very often fail to cooperate with each other.

Many cultures are fragmented on the basis of ethnicity, and utilization of health services is closely related to the existence of ethnic sub-cultures. Israel has one of the highest utilization rates in the world. In an explanation of this, Shuval et al.[13] have noted that the Israeli health-care-delivery system, as a result of the nature of the consumer, the sick role, the social structure of the medical institutions, and the social system of the larger society, performs latent functions in addition to manifest ones. This concern with latent functions is unique, and it has created a focus on nonmedical needs such as those related to catharsis, coping with failure, integration into Israeli society, status, and the resolution of a magic-science conflict. In addition, Margolis attributes the need to perform many of these latent functions to the decline of Zionist ideology, along with the existence of ethnic subcultures.[14]

Moreover, ethnicity can be related to treatment. For example, it accounted for Fanon's self-admitted failure in Algeria in that he attempted to integrate Moslem and European therapy. Also one can cite the practice of herbal medicine today, especially in Hispanic and Indian cultures.

Ideology not only influences health policy and the structure of the delivery system but its functions as well as medical care and medical practice. Gibson, using China as a case study, aptly notes that through system input of ideological information, social control over a key professional area is maintained, He argues that ideology has an impact on the functional prerequisites of the health-care system as they concern goal attainment, adaptation, integration, and tension management. He specifically cites the significance of ideology as a guide to technical details involving diagnostic and therapeutic decision making.[15] Also one may note that much of the same holds true for the Soviet Union where the practice of medicine in general and psychiatry in particular is closely related to ideology. In that nation medicine is utilized as an instrument of governmental control.

There are many aspects of political culture that relate to health. Given space limitations, only some of the most general have been presented here. Other economic and demographic concepts that include aggregate-data variables might be discussed along with certain sociological variables such as the character of the social stratification system, and so on. However, it should be pointed out that there is disagreement concerning the appropriateness of these variables to the concept of political culture.[16] Although many of the examples cited in this chapter are frequently considered in the nations mentioned, their relation to cultural values is not always undertaken. Political culture, being a collective property of groups such as nations, subnational units, or social groupings, is useful to students of health care for comparative purposes. It can be used to link the micro and macro levels of analysis and to explain differences and similarities among collectivities. Furthermore, it allows for an understanding of the political process in the health-care sector.

> This perspective highlights the context in which the life of politics and the politics of life take place. The values and social arrangements of every society create biases that favor some interests, promote certain courses of action, and determine whether some issues and policy options get on the political agenda at all . . . . this approach can reveal new alternatives, identify probable consequences of policy choice, and, in explaining some policy patterns, suggest the limits of public policy intervention.[17]

Moreover, political culture can be used in an explanation of the actual operation of the health care delivery system. Using political culture as a tool of analysis one can seek to understand why collectivities possess different health care delivery arrangements, why these institutions operate in various modes and why actors within the system and those served by it hold certain beliefs and behave in a particular way. In a sense, political culture serves as a perceptual screen which determines how one views or comprehends a specific set of circumstances, or a particular set of institutions.[18] However, as an explanatory tool, political culture must be used in conjunction with other closely related types of explanations whether they be structural, institutional, or functional. The utility of political culture as an explanatory instrument lies in the fact that it can be complemented by other variables.

Obviously, too often political culture is approached as a static notion when, in reality, it is a constantly changing phenomenon. Extensive research in political development and mobilization has made this evident. In dealing with the dynamic element, the agents of socialization that transmit political-culture values must be carefully examined and utilized where possible in terms of providing the appropriate setting for improvement in health care. The process of development is affected by the political culture as well as the nature of the various socializing agents. Thus utilization of political culture as an analytic tool affords one a better comprehension of the policies and necessary investments in various socializing agents that can best produce the desired health-care-delivery system.

In spite of its limitations, the concept of political culture represents a significant dimension of the comparative study of the delivery of health services.

Notes

1. Gabriel A. Almond and Sidney Verba, *The Civic Culture: Political Attitudes and Democracy in Five Nations* (Boston: Little, Brown, 1965), pp. 13-14.

2. Hirobumi Ito, "Health Insurance Policy Development in Denmark and Sweden: 1860-1950," *Social Science and Medicine* 13c(October 1979):143-160.

3. David Elkins and Richard E.B. Simeon, "A Cause in Search of Its Effect, or What Does Political Culture Explain?" *Comparative Politics* 11 (January 1979):131.

4. Giuseppe Di Palma, "Institutional Rules and Legislative Outcomes in the Italian Parliament," *Legislative Studies Quarterly* 1(1976):147-179.

5. Richard M. Titmuss, *The Gift Relationship: From Human Blood to Social Policy* (London: George Allen and Unwin Ltd., 1971).

6. *British Record*, 16 August 1975, pp. 3-4.

7. Giacomo Sani, "The Political Culture of Italy: Continuity and Change," in *The Civic Culture Revisited*, edited by Gabriel A. Almond and Sidney Verba (Boston: Little, Brown, 1980), pp. 308-310.

8. For example, see Sondra Z. Koff, "Emergency Medical Services in a Rural Setting: Attitudes of Policy-Makers and Consumers," *Journal of Health and Human Resources Administration,* forthcoming.

9. William C. Stratmann et al., "A Study of Consumer Attitudes about Health Care: The Control, Cost and Financing of Health Services," *Medical Care* 13(August 1975):668.

10. Margaret A. Peisert and David M. Stevens, "The Illinois Emergency Medical Services System: Public Knowledge, Attitudes and Utilization." (Paper presented at the 104th American Public Health Association Annual Meeting, Miami Beach, 20 October 1976), p. 7.

11. William E. Bertrand, "Attitudinal Classification of Health Manpower in Columbia: A Research Note on Urban/Rural Differences in Occupational Prestige," *Social Science and Medicine* 13A (March 1979):235-240.

12. John D. Hutcheson, Jr. and George A. Taylor, "Religious Variables, Political System Characteristics, and Policy Outputs in the American States," *American Journal of Political Science*, XVII(1973), 414-421.

13. Judith T. Shuval et al., *Social Functions of Medical Practice* (San Francisco: Jossey-Bass, 1970).

14. Emmanuel Margolis, "Health Care in a Changing Society: The Health Services of Israel," *Medical Care* 13(November 1975):944.

15. Geoffrey Gibson, "Chinese Medical Practice and the Thoughts of Chairman Mao," *Social Science and Medicine* 6(1972):67-93.

16. Lawrence C. Mayer, *Comparative Political Inquiry: A Methodological Survey* (Homewood, Ill.: The Dorsey Press, 1972), p. 169.

17. Theodore R. Marmor and Amy Bridges, "Introduction to Special Issue: Politics, Medicine and Health," *Journal of Health Politics, Policy and Law* 4(Fall 1979):355.

18. Elkins and Simeon "A Cause in Search of Its Effect," pp. 139-140.

14 International Comparisons of Health Services: How? Who? Why?

Victor W. Sidel

There is increasing use of comparisons with health services in other societies to sharpen understanding of problems in our own health services and to attempt to find models for constructive change.[1] Such comparisons, however, often raise methodologic and conceptual questions—about the validity of the data, their analysis, and their applicability to our own situation—that are as difficult to deal with as the service-related problems the comparisons are meant to illuminate. These questions include the choice of methods of comparison, identification of observer biases, and most important, definition of the purpose of the comparison: horizon expanding? paradigm smashing? question defining? model seeking? pitfall avoiding? inspiration giving? The point of this chapter is that if the observer does not clearly examine and address—in data collection, analysis, and form of presentation—the nature and the purpose of the comparison, the effort may produce a fascinating travelogue or an elegant pedantic exercise but will not help provoke and guide useful change.

How?—Methods for International Comparisons of Health Services

Descriptive Methods

By Insiders. Some of the most valuable insights into the health services of a society come, of course, from knowledgeable people within it. In general, those working and living within a society have enormous advantages over outside observers in their depth and breadth of experience with the system, with its nuances, and with its regional variations. Conversely, insiders—unless they have extensive knowledge of relevant systems in other societies—may have great difficulty in isolating and describing those elements of their system that are of greatest comparative interest. Furthermore, insiders are usually enmeshed

This chapter is based in part on a presentation by the author in the session, "Occupational Health and Safety: An International Perspective" at the Annual Meeting of the American Public Health Association, New York City, November 1979.

in the social, cultural, economic, and political structure of their own society; bottom-dwelling fish, it has been argued, would be the last ones to take any special notice of water because it is all around them all the time. Finally, many insiders may fear personal loss from certain types of description of the system in which they work, if the description or its purposes are viewed negatively by those who control their jobs or the system itself.

A special problem in the use of descriptions by insiders arises when the descriptions do not make clear the unique conditions prevailing within the society. For example, many current descriptions by Chinese observers of the impact of the "Gang of Four" on health services are based on the presumption of knowledge of the structure of their society, of the metaphorical language being used, and of the range of issues that are included in (and, more important, excluded from) the debate. When the descriptions are presented to a foreign visitor to China or read outside China, they may take on a meaning quite unintended by the describer and quite at variance with what actually occurred.[2]

By Outsiders. Outsiders have the important advantage of knowing which elements of the system being analyzed for comparison are of greatest relevance to their own or other societies. Outsiders can express descriptions in language that is more comprehensible and focused for people at home. Outsiders often (but certaintly not always) have less to lose from negative description of the system they are visiting and less to gain from flattery of those controlling it. Amphibians, in short, take special note of the water because they are aware, from personal experience, that some species live outside it. Outsiders, to use another clichéd example, may be able to see the forest while insiders are looking at trees.

But, outsiders' descriptions are of course also limited. Observations by outsiders will almost certainly have to be more superficial than those of insiders. Furthermore, outsiders may be more likely than insiders to generalize inappropriately to an entire society from the examples observed, while insiders know how varied the trees are. There are surely comparative advantages in describing the whole forest—which insiders may be unable to do effectively because the regional variations seem so enormous—but only if the signficant variations are also described.[3]

Statistical Methods

Compilation of Existing Statistics. The limitations of descriptive methods have led many concerned with international comparisons to concentrate rather on what they view as "hard" data, statistics on health services and on health status that have already been collected or that they can collect within each society. Insofar as the statistics are based on common, easily understandable definitions and are collected in comparable ways, such comparisons may be very useful. At one end of the spectrum, for example. "death"—despite some problems of definition in a very few patients at the instant of dying—is quite easy to define and gathering data on numbers of deaths in most industrialized countries is relatively easy; it is difficult in such countries to hid the fact of a death from public data-gathering agencies and deaths are therefore reliably counted and aggregated. In poor countries, of course, formal reporting of death may not be so universal nor data collection and aggregation so routine, but crude death rates are usually reasonably valid. Going beyond simple gross numbers of deaths, however, to more refined measures—cause-specific mortality rates, for example—brings great problems of comparability even among industrialized countries. Whether suicide, to choose a particularly difficult cause to pin down, is listed on the death certificate depends on a multitude of factors including the social or religious stigma and/or the economic loss that accrues to the family of a suicide victim, the sensitivity and knowledge of the person making out the certificate and the ways in which the certificates are designed, safeguarded against breach of confidentiality, and analyzed. Moving further, from mortality statistics to morbidity statistics, of course, greatly magnifies the problems of comparability; for certain diseases such as "mental illness," routinely collected data are almost useless for intercultural or international comparison.

The advantages and disadvantages in the use of statistical data on health status are also found in the use of statistical data on health services. This is true whether one is dealing with structure (for example, numbers of doctors or hospital beds per capita) or process (for example, numbers of patient visits or hospitalizations per capita). Surely, knowing and comparing hard data in these areas is extremely useful in comparing health services. Equally surely, definitions of "doctors" and of "hospital beds," of "visits" and of "hospitalizations," differ among societies and particularly differ between industrialized and developing countries. This is not to say that important impressions cannot be derived from imperfect statistical data. Rather, those who decry descriptive data and allege that only statistical data are valid for comparisons may be misleading themselves and others.

Collection of Statistical Data by Standardized Cross-National Surveys. Problems with routinely gathered statistical data have led to increasing attempts in recent years to perform structured, standardized surveys simultaneously in a number of societies. Elaborate methods have been developed, for example, for translating and back-translating survey instruments and for standardized training of surveyors. Some major surveys, covering a range of countries and a range of topics, have been extremely expensive—in human resources, in money, and in opportunity costs. An example is the World Health Organization/International Collaborative Study of Medical Care Utilization[4]; the study was conducted by

"90 professional workers supported by about 300 technical personnel" over a 12-year period in selected areas in seven countries.

In my opinion, the returns on many of these major investments have been modest. My reason for saying this is not only that the range of data collected and the geographic sample within each country, despite great effort, is usually very narrow and may be unrepresentative. More important, data gathered at such great effort and cost may be accorded an influence in comparison that goes beyond their value, part of a general tendency to treat parameters for which hard data are available as more important than those for which the data are soft. This is the problem that Alfred North Whitehead, in quite another context, described as the "fallacy of misplaced concreteness."

In addition to these problems with statistical data, there is the temptation, once the hard data are in hand, to omit the next step, of tying them to the special conditions—often known only descriptively—in the country in which they were collected. A classic example of a problem in the interpretation of such data is provided by an international study of sick-absence rates in industry. The data, summarized in the first column of table 14-1, showed a wide range of sick-absence rates in the countries studied. The temptation would be to use these data to compare health and illness, or even to compare the effectiveness of health services in these societies. However, as the author who presented the data pointed out, there is a remarkably strong inverse correlation between sick-absence rates and unemployment rates. The interpretation of the hard comparative data on sick-absence is therefore complex. The low rates may be due to greater fear of losing a job in countries with high unemployment; as a middle-class respondent in Koos' *Health of Regionville* put it, "How do you know when you're sick, anyway? Some people can go to bed most any time with anything, but most of us can't be sick—even when we need to be."[5] Another explanation,

Table 14-1
Relationship of Sick-Absence Rate to Unemployment Rate

	Sick-Absence Rate, 1956[a]	Unemployment Rate, 1960
Federal Republic of Germany	5.7	1.0
Sweden	5.6	1.5
France	4.6	1.9
United Kingdom	4.3	2.4
Italy	2.6	4.3
United States	1.9	5.6
Canada	1.1	7.0

Source: Adapted from Philip Enterline, "Sick Absence in Certain Western Countries," *Industrial Medicine and Surgery* 33(October 1964):738-774.

[a]Percentage of employed persons absent from work on an average day due to illness.

not incompatible with the first, is that in countries of high unemployment, employers have a larger pool of workers to choose from and are therefore able to choose healthier workers or at least workers less likely to be absent. Whatever the explanation of the variation, simple reliance on the sick-absence data—even though definitions are clear and data collection excellent—to draw conclusions about health status or health services would be misleading.

Choice of Countries for Comparison. Perhaps the most significant way in which the methods for international comparison of health services affect the results is in the selection of countries for comparison. Although the selection may at times appear opportunistic (based on availability of data or on opportunities for travel) or even random, I believe this is rarely the case. Observers generally create opportunities for travel or collaboration and select or ignore available data from large numbers of choices. Since there are few widely accepted standards for choosing systems for comparison—in contrast to standards for comparability of statistical data, which exist but are often ignored—the observer usually selects those societies for comparison that will make the desired point.[6]

Who?—People Performing International Comparisons of Health Services

Roles within the System

The perceptions of anyone studying a health-care system, whether the observer's own or a foreign one, whether the method is descriptive or statistical, will be colored by the role the observer plays within his or her own system. The important differences in perception of quality of health-care services between providers and consumers of them have been repeatedly demonstrated. But even within these broad groups there are great differences. Among the providers, doctors, nurses, social workers, laboratory technicians, maintenance workers, administrators, and planners—to name only a few—will have very diverse ways of observing and describing a system or choosing which statistics are most valid for comparison. Among the consumers, social class, race, level of education, location of residence, and health status (and, if ill, whether the illness is acute or chronic) will all enter—consciously or unconsciously, perceptibly or imperceptibly—into the analysis.[7]

Perceptions of the Nature of Society

Distinct from the impact of the observer's role within the system, the observer also approaches any analysis of that role in the context of a world view. There are, for example, physicians in the United States who view their experience in the context of the philosophy of Ayn Rand[8] and others who bring to it the insights of Karl Marx.[9] Any comparative study must reflect, in one way or another, the underlying social philosophy of the observer. One observer is likely to be more concerned with issues of freedom of choice and with conditions of professional work; the other with the impact of the system on equity, on what is perceived as justice for the least advantaged within the society. The concerns and insights of the observer, needless to add, will profoundly affect the selection of data and their analysis.

Why?—Reasons for Performing International Comparisons of Health Services

Raising Questions about One's Own System

One of the most common reasons for entering into a comparative study is to raise questions about one's own system, to use the experiences of others as a mirror against which to view the successes or failures of the system at home. The questions raised may be broad or narrow, including expanding the horizons of the reader ("health care really can be provided very differently"), exposing the assumptions on which the reader's own system is based ("there are quite different paradigms for health and illness in other cultures"), or raising doubts about specific practices ("why must it be done that way?").[10]

Seeking Alternative Models for Care

The point of the comparison may go beyond raising questions about one's own system to the suggestion that another society's system—or elements of it—may be models worthy of emulation. Clearly, since a health-care system is a reflection and component of a society's cultural, social, political, and economic conditions, such suggestions must be carefully stated and appropriately limited. Even when the model suggested for emulation is a narrow technical one, the nature of the broader system or of the society in which it is embedded must be considered; for example, data showing that heart-attack victims in Great Britain do as well when cared for at home as they do when hospitalized must be viewed in the context of the British National Health Service's capability for caring for people at home, a capability unmatched by the systems of many other industrialized countries.

Avoiding the Pitfalls in Other Systems

This is the mirror image of the previous point, but it is of interest that those who use comparisons to point out failures in other systems rarely note that the same care must be used in identifying models for avoidance as for identifying models for emulation. Rarely is it pointed out that failures of a system, like its successes, may be a product of very different social and economic conditions.[11]

Finding Inspiration in the Efforts of Other Societies

Since all significant social change that is designed to benefit those who have the least wealth and power in a society requires struggle against those who now have wealth and power and seek to hold onto it, comparisons with other societies may be used to point out that some have indeed been able to produce such changes in health services. Much that has been written about services in revolutionary societies such as China, Cuba, and Tanzania is intended—directly or indirectly—to make this point; at times analyses of health service in these societies are used to make the further point that significant changes in power structure may be necessary in order to permit significant changes in the structure of health services and, conversely, that local efforts to change health services may contribute to the broader struggle to change the locus of power in the society.[12]

So What?—The Responsibility of Those Who Attempt International Comparisons of Health Services

If comparisons are to be used to help bring about useful change, those who would do so must recognize some of the pitfalls as well as advantages of using them. If the methods and their biases, the observers and their biases, and—most important of all—the purposes and their underlying assumptions, are not clearly identified in the comparison, the reader or listener is likely to be misled, turned off, or both. This is not to say, on the one hand, that polemics or travelogues, which almost by definition lack these niceties, cannot be useful in influencing change. At the other extreme, academic reports that emphasize the limitations in the data and the analysis to the point that effective communication of the ideas is impeded may be useless. In the middle, explicit identification of the methods and the purposes underlying the comparison if the comparison itself is relevant and clearly drawn, will make it more convincing and effective.

Another reason for clear recognition of the problems of international comparisons of health and health services is the special context of such studies.

Data from international comparisons are likely to be deeply misleading and are at best useless without a clear understanding by the audience of the social, political, economic and cultural conditions in which they are embedded. These conditions are, at root, the determinants of the health status of the population and of the structure and function of the health services. Consideration of data on health or health services without consideration, for example, of the power structure of the society, of the extent to which health services are used to redistribute wealth and power, of the ways in which health services contribute to or detract from community life, of the uses of health services as instruments of social control, of the burden of the direct and indirect costs of health services, and of the coherence between health services and the cultural traditions of those served. The determinants of health and of health services, in short, are predominantly social, and those who compare health services transnationally have a responsibility to make this relationship clear.

The final reason for clarity about methods and purpose for those who would compare health systems is to guide their work. The choices of societies for comparison are so numerous—and the range of elements available for comparison so broad—that without such clarity the effort is unlikely to be successful. Since resources for international studies are limited and opportunity costs great, clear understanding of purpose and method are indispensable for those who believe that analysis and change go hand in hand, that the purpose of international comparisons in health is not only to understand the world but to change it.[13]

Notes

1. Extensive bibliographies of such studies may be found in R. Kohn and S. Radius, "International Comparison of Health Services Systems," *International Journal of Health Services* 3(2)(1973):295-309; Jesus DeMiguel, "A Framework for the Study of National Health Systems," *Inquiry* Supplement 12(2)(June 1975):10-24; and in many of the sources listed below.

2. See, for example, The Criticism Group of the Ministry of Health, "Conspiracy of the 'Gang of Four' to Usurp Party and State Power in Health Departments," *Chinese Medical Journal*, New Series, 3(July 1977):213-217; this was in part a response to Miao Yu, "Beat Back Right Deviationist Wind on Medical and Health Front," *Chinese Medical Journal*, New Series, 2(July 1976):231-236. A similar problem occurs when socialist supporters of the British National Health Service, attempting to make it more equitable by highlighting its remaining maldistributions, fail to emphasize for foreign readers the extent to which it has provided fairer distribution and equity; see, for example, Julian Tudor Hart, "The Inverse Care Law," *The Lancet* 1(1973):611-616 and Vicente Navarro, *Class Struggle, the State, and Medicine* (PRODIST, 1978).

3. An example of a book on international comparisons in health based entirely on descriptions by insiders is I. Douglas-Wilson and Gordon McLachlan, eds., *Health Service Prospects: An International Survey* (Little, Brown, 1973). An example of a descriptive book written entirely by an outsider is Milton Roemer, *Health Care Systems in World Perspective* (Health Administration Press, 1976); it covers 45 countries on all the continents. Examples of materials that combine inside and outside descriptions are Roemer's *Social Medicine* (Springer Publishing, 1978); Kenneth Newell, ed., *Health by the People* (World Health Organization, 1975); Vicente Navarro, *Medicine under Capitalism* (PRODIST, 1976); and Victor Sidel and Ruth Sidel, *A Healthy State: An International Perspective on the Crisis in U.S. Medical Care* (Pantheon Books, 1978).

4. The methods for the study are described in "Use of Health Care: An International Study," *WHO Chronicle* 30 (October 1976): 403-406. The full study was published as Robert Kohn and Kerr White, eds., *Health Care: An International Study* (London: Oxford University Press, 1976); a summary is Kerr White, "International Comparisons of Medical Care," *Scientific American* 233(2)(August 1975):17-25. Another, much more limited example is Mitchell Balter, Jerome Levine, and Dean Manheimer, "Cross-national Study of the Extent of Anti-Anxiety Sedative Drug Use," *New England Journal of Medicine* 290(14)(4 April 1974):769-774.

5. Earl Koos, *The Health of Regionville* (Hafner Publishing, 1954), p. 30.

6. An attempt to establish criteria for selection of systems for comparison was made in Roy Elling and Henry Kerr, "Selection of Contrasting Health Systems for In-Depth Study," *Inquiry,* Supplement 12(2)(June 1975):25-40.

7. Some of the differences in perception between physicians and patients and their consequences for planning are discussed in Victor Sidel, "Quality for Whom? Effects of Professional Responsibility for Quality of Health Care on Equity," *Bulletin of the New York Academy of Medicine* 52(January 1976): 164-177.

8. For example, Robert Sade, "Medical Care as a Right: A Refutation," *New England Journal of Medicine* 285(2 December 1971):1288-1292.

9. For example, Howard Waitzkin, "A Marxist View of Medical Care," *Annals of Internal Medicine* 89(August 1978):264-278.

10. See, for example, Sander Kelman, "The Social Nature of the Definition Problem in Health," *International Journal of Health Services* 5(4)(1975):625-642.

11. This failure to clarify the nature of the comparison at times seems purposeful, as in the publication by the American Medical Association of *The British Health Care System* (AMA, 1976) and by Roche Laboratories of Cotton Lindsay, *National Health Issues: The British Experience* (Hoffman-LaRoche, 1980), both of which, for obvious reasons, magnify the flaws of the British National Health Service.

12. See, for example, Victor Sidel and Ruth Sidel, *Serve the People:*

Observations on Medicine in the People's Republic of China (Beacon Press, 1974); S. Guttmacher and R. Danielson, "Changes in Cuban Health Care: An Argument against Technological Pessimism," *International Journal of Health Services* 7(1977):383-400; and Oscar Gish, *Planning the Health Sector: The Tanzanian Experience* (Croom, Helm, Ltd., 1975); similar points are made in the chapters on these countries in Kenneth Newell, ed., *Health by the People*.

13. Two excellent annotated bibliographies on international comparisons of health services have been compiled by Professor Ray H. Elling of the University of Connecticut, and both bibliographies were published by the Gale Research Company of Detroit, Michigan, in 1980. They are *Cross-National Study of Health Systems: Countries, World Regions, and Special Problems— A Guide to Information Sources* and *Cross-National Study of Health Systems: Concepts, Methods, and Data Sources—A Guide to Information Sources.*

Index of Names

185

Index of Subjects

List of Contributors

James M. Cameron is assistant professor of public health, School of Public Health, University of California, Los Angeles.

Jon B. Christianson is associate professor, Department of Economics and Department of Public Policy, Planning, and Administration, University of Arizona.

Mark R. Daniels is assistant professor of political science, Department of Political Science, Oklahoma State University.

Raisa B. Deber is assistant professor, Department of Health Administration and Department of Political Economy, University of Toronto.

David Falcone is associate professor of health administration and political science, Department of Health Administration, Duke University.

Joseph L. Falkson is president and chief executive officer of Health Sector Management, Inc., in Washington, D.C.

Steven Jonas is associate professor of community and preventive medicine, School of Medicine, State University of New York at Stony Brook.

Louanne Kennedy is assistant professor, Department of Health Care Administration at Bernard M. Baruch College–Mt. Sinai School of Medicine, The City University of New York.

Sondra Z. Koff is associate professor of political science, State University of New York at Binghamton.

Walter McClure is vice-president and director of health policy and planning for InterStudy, an independent policy-research organization located in Minneapolis, Minnesota.

Joseph C. Morreale is associate professor of economics, Bard College.

James L. Regens is assistant professor of political science, University of Georgia.

Elianne Riska is associate professor, Department of Sociology and College of Human Medicine, Michigan State University.

Victor W. Sidel is professor and chairperson, Department of Social Medicine, Montefiore Hospital and Medical Center, Albert Einstein College of Medicine.

Deborah A. Stone is associate professor of political science, Massachusetts Institute of Technology.

About the Editors

Ralph A. Straetz is professor of health policy, Department of Politics, New York University. He was one of the first political scientists to work in the field of health and mental-health policy. A founding member of the Committee on Health Politics, he has been its chairman for ten years. Professor Straetz directed a Ph.D. research training program in mental-health policy funded by the National Institute of Mental Health and a similar program sponsored by the National Center for Health Services Research. He is founding editor of *Journal of Health Politics, Policy and Law.*

Marvin Lieberman is executive secretary of the Committee on Medicine in Society of New York Academy of Medicine. He is a graduate of The City College of New York, and received the Ph.D. in politics from New York University School of Law. He was formerly associate director of the program in political science and health policy at New York University. Dr. Lieberman has taught at Rutgers University and is currently an adjunct faculty member at the New School for Social Research and Sarah Lawrence College. He has done research and has published articles on the financing of mental-illness services, legal and ethical issues in occupational safety and health, and on the organization of health care.

Alice Sardell is assistant professor in the Department of Urban Studies at Queens College, The City University of New York. She received the Ph.D. in politics from New York University where she was a Fellow in political science and health policy research. She has published articles on health policy and on the welfare-rights movement. Her current research is on the politics of ambulatory care.